LIBRARY TECHNOLOGY FOR VISUALLY AND PHYSICALLY IMPAIRED PATRONS

Supplements to
COMPUTERS IN LIBRARIES

1. Essential Guide to dBase III+ in Libraries
   Karl Beiser
   ISBN 0-88736-064-5   1987
2. Essential Guide to Bulletin Board Systems
   Patrick R. Dewey
   ISBN 0-88736-066-1   1987
3. Microcomputers for the Online Searcher
   Ralph Alberico
   ISBN 0-88736-093-9   1987
4. Printers for Use with OCLC Workstations
   James Speed Hensinger
   ISBN 0-88736-180-3   1987
5. Developing Microcomputer Work Areas in Academic Libraries
   Jeannine Uppgard
   ISBN 0-88736-233-8   1988
6. Microcomputers and the Reference Librarian
   Patrick R. Dewey
   ISBN 0-88736-234-6   1988
7. Retrospective Conversion: A Practical Guide for Libraries
   Jane Beaumont and Joseph P. Cox
   ISBN 0-88736-352-0   1988
8. Connecting with Technology 1988: Microcomputers in Libraries
   Nancy Melin Nelson, ed.
   ISBN 0-88736-330-X   1989
9. The Macintosh ® Press: Desktop Publishing for Libraries
   Richard D. Johnson and Harriett H. Johnson
   ISBN 0-88736-287-7   1989
10. Expert Systems for Reference and Information Retrieval
    Ralph Alberico and Mary Micco
    ISBN 0-88736-232-X   1990
11. EMail for Libraries
    Patrick R. Dewey
    ISBN 0-88736-327-X   1989
12. 101 Uses of dBase in Libraries
    Lynne Hayman, ed.
    ISBN 0-88736-427-6   1990
13. FAX for Libraries
    Patrick R. Dewey
    ISBN 0-88736-480-2   1990
14. The Librarian's Guide to WordPerfect 5.0
    Cynthia LaPier
    ISBN 0-88736-493-4   1990
15. Technology for the 90's
    Nancy Melin Nelson, ed.
    ISBN 0-88736-487-X   1990
16. Microcomputer Management and Maintenance for Libraries
    Elizabeth S. Lane
    ISBN 0-88736-522-1   1990
17. Public Access CD-ROMs in Libraries: Case Studies
    Linda Stewart, Kathy Chiang, and Bill Coons, eds.
    ISBN 0-88736-516-7   1990
18. The Systems Librarian Guide to Computers
    Michael Schuyler and Elliott Swanson
    ISBN 0-88736-580-9   1990
19. Essential Guide to dBase IV in Libraries
    Karl Beiser
    ISBN 0-88736-530-2   1991
20. UNIX and Libraries
    D. Scott Brandt
    ISBN 0-88736-541-8   1991
21. Integrated Online Library Catalogs
    Jennifer Cargill, ed.
    ISBN 0-88736-675-9   1990
22. CD-ROM Retrieval Software: An Overview
    Blaine Victor Morrow
    ISBN 0-88736-667-8   1991
23. CD-ROM Licensing and Copyright Issues for Libraries
    Meta Nissley and Nancy Melin Nelson, editors
    ISBN 0-88736-701-1   1990
24. CD-ROM Local Area Networks: A User's Guide
    Norman Desmarais, ed.
    ISBN 0-88736-700-3   1991
25. Library Technology 1970-1990: Shaping the Library of the Future
    Nancy Melin Nelson, ed.
    ISBN 0-88736-695-3   1991
26. Library Technology for Visually and Physically Impaired Patrons
    Barbara T. Mates
    ISBN 0-88736-704-6   1991
27. Local Area Networks in Libraries
    Kenneth Marks and Steven Nielsen
    ISBN 0-88736-705-4   1991
28. Small Project Automation for Libraries and Information Centers
    Jane Mandelbaum
    ISBN 0-88736-731-3   1991
29. Text Management for Libraries and Information Centers: Tools and Techniques
    Erwin K. Welsch and Kurt F. Welsch
    ISBN 0-88736-737-2   1992
30. Library Systems Migration: Changing Automated Systems in Libraries and Information Centers
    Gary M. Pitkin, ed.
    ISBN 0-88736-738-0   1991
31. From A - Z39.50: A Networking Primer
    James J. Michael
    ISBN 0-88736-766-6   1992
32. Search Sheets for OPACs on the Internet
    Marcia Henry, Linda Keenan, Michael Reagan
    ISBN 0-88736-767-4   1991
33. Directory of Directories on the Internet
    Ray Metz
    ISBN 0-88736-768-2   1991
34. Building Blocks for the National Network: Initiatives and Individuals
    Nancy Melin Nelson
    ISBN 0-88736-769-0   1991
35. Public Institutions: Capitalizing on the Internet
    Charles Worsley
    ISBN 0-88736-770-4   1991
36. A Directory of Computer Conferencing for Libraries
    Brian Williams
    ISBN 0-88736-771-2   1991
37. Optical Character Recognition: A Librarian's Guide
    Marlene Ogg and Harold Ogg
    ISBN 0-88736-778-X   1991
38. CD-ROM Research Collections
    Pat Ensor
    ISBN 0-88736-779-8   1991
39. Library LANs: Case Studies in Practice and Application
    Marshall Breeding
    ISBN 0-88736-786-0   1992
40. 101 Uses of Spreadsheets in Libraries
    Robert Machalow
    ISBN 0-88736-791-7   1992
41. Library Computing in Canada: Bilingualism, Multiculturalism, and Transborder Connections
    Nancy Melin Nelson and Eric Flower, eds.
    ISBN 0-88736-792-5   1991
42. CD-ROM in Libraries: A Reader
    Meta Nissley, ed.
    ISBN 0-88736-800-X   1992
43. Automating the Library with AskSam: A Practical Handbook
    Marcia D. Talley and Virginia A. McNitt
    ISBN 0-88736-801-8   1991
44. The Evolution of Library Automation: Management Issues and Future Perspectives
    Gary M. Pitkin, editor
    ISBN 0-88736-811-5   1991

LIBRARY TECHNOLOGY FOR VISUALLY AND PHYSICALLY IMPAIRED PATRONS

Barbara T. Mates

Meckler
Westport • London

Library of Congress Cataloging-in-Publication Data

Mates, Barbara T.
   Library technology for visually and physically impaired patrons / Barbara T. Mates.
      p.   cm. -- (Supplements to Computers in libraries ; 26)
   Includes bibliographical references and index.
   ISBN 0-88736-704-6 : $
   1. Libraries and the visually handicapped. 2. Libraries and the physically handicapped. 3. Library science--Technological innovations. 4. Physically handicapped--Services for. 5. Visually handicapped--Services for. 6. Information technology.
7. Libraries--Automation.   I. Title.   II. Series.
Z711.92V57M37   1991
027.6'63--dc20   91-31056
                                                CIP

British Library Cataloguing-in-Publication Data

Mates, Barbara T.
Library technology for visually and physically impaired patrons. - (Supplements to computers in libraries)
I. Title II. Series
027.6

ISBN 0-88736-704-6

Copyright © 1991 Meckler Publishing. All rights reserved. No part of this publication may be reproduced in any form by any means without prior written permission from the publisher, except by a reviewer who may quote brief passages in review.

Meckler Publishing, the publishing division of Meckler Corporation,
   11 Ferry Lane West, Westport, CT 06880.
Meckler Ltd., 247-249 Vauxhall Bridge Road,
   London SW1V 1HQ, U.K.

Printed on acid free paper.
Printed and bound in the United States of America.

This book is dedicated to my parents, Ann and (the late) Anthony Trask, in appreciation of the sacrifices they made with love, to insure my growth and education.

And to my husband, James, for his love, patience, understanding and encouragement.

Contents

Preface and Acknowledgments ix

   1. Technology and the Disabled—Surveying Your Needs 1
   2. Large-Print Access 11
   3. Braille Access 27
   4. Audio Output 47
   5. Optical Character Recognition (OCR) Systems 63
   6. Keyboards 71
   7. Processing Information Without a Keyboard 83
   8. Technology to Assist the Deaf and Hearing Impaired 107
   9. Putting Technology to Work in Your Library 115
  10. Future Growth of Adaptive Technology 139

Appendix 1: Registered Readers (Thousands) of the NLS Network 145
Appendix 2: Vendors and Distributors of Technological Devices for the
            Blind and Physically Handicapped 146
Appendix 3: CD-ROM Titles that Translate into Special Format 154
Appendix 4: Bulletin Boards Addressing Handicapped Person's Needs 155
Appendix 5: Funding Sources for Adaptive Equipment 157
Notes 159
Glossary 169
Bibliography 173
General Index 181
Product/Vendor Index 185

Preface and Acknowledgments

Offering specialized library services for the visually and physically impaired has always been a debated topic. While professionals and politicians agree that this group of people is entitled to library service, they are quick to point out that adaptive devices are too expensive for such a small group and that visually or physically impaired patrons should be referred to one of the 55 Regional Libraries for the Blind and Physically Handicapped of the National Library Service (NLS) Network, established in 1932.[1] Acknowledging the fact that the Regional Library approach is the only way to economically and efficiently provide vast amounts of recreational reading material to the masses, it is not the answer for the traditional reference service which requires answers to questions in a timely fashion. While some of the network libraries do offer visually impaired people a place to go to read their own correspondence, they are not required to and many are miles away from the people who need the services.

Recent technology has finally made it economically feasible for public and academic libraries to provide services beyond recreational reading to persons needing reference access and services in special media such as braille, large print and voice output, and to provide magnifying devices for a quickly aging population.

It is the "ready" or "quick" reference service that has been missing from library service. Recording for the Blind,[2] located in Princeton, New Jersey, provides educational, vocational, and supplemental general interest materials, as well as text-books, but is still unable to provide the information that is found in a general reference department of a print library. Within the last few years a few of the NLS Regional Libraries, "special needs" centers as well as some public and academic libraries have taken advantage of technology and provided their patrons with access to a wealth of previously denied information.

The majority of the libraries, however, have been able to give information in regular print to all, but people needing the information in braille are reluctant to take advantage of the wealth on the reference shelves simply because they would need someone to translate it for them. Patrons who must depend on a sighted reader to read bank statements and other essential correspondence hesitate to ask someone to read them a page from the *World Almanac*, simply because they are curious about a topic. What this means is that a print-impaired person could not look up basic information on a Middle-East country or trace a congressman's voting record on any given issue.

x *Preface and Acknowledgments*

The last decade saw the refinement of the personal computer and peripherals as well as the development of the CD-ROM. Although not specifically designed to aid the disabled, these advancements (with adaptions) are enabling the disabled population to access and assimilate virtually any title on disc (either CD-ROM disc or PC diskette). Figure 1 illustrates the dramatic growth of accessible ready reference sources to the visually and physically impaired by CD-ROM.

BRAILLE	CASSETTE	LARGE PRINT	
HANDY GRAMMAR REFERENCE WORLD BOOK			1959
GERRISH TEC. DIC. ROGET'S THES. WEBSTER'S NEW WORLD DICT.	ELEMENTS OF STYLE	WORLD BOOK	1969
WRITERS HAND BOOK	CONCISE HER. DICT. M-H HANDBOOK OF ENGLISH MERCK MANUAL	AMERICN HER. DICT. COMPTON'S SCI. CONST. OF THE U.S. MERR-WEB DICT. & THESAURUS	1979
BARTLETT'S QUOTATIONS CONSTITUTION PDR		AFTER 50 PHAR. COLUMBIA CONC. ENCYCLOPEDIA HAMMONDS WORLD ATLAS ISIS LG. PRT. DICTIONARY	1980
CONSTITUTION PAPERS GROLIER'S E.E. M-H ENC. OF SCI. & TECH. MICROSOFT BKS. PDR	CONSTITUTION PAPERS GROLIER'S E.E. M-H ENC. OF SCI. & TECH. MICROSOFT BKS.	CONSTITUTION PAPERS GROLIER'S E.E. M-H ENC. OF SCI. & TECH. PDR	1989
WORD CRUNCHER WORLD FACT BK. U.S. HIST. ON CD-ROM LIBRARY OF THE FUTURE	WORD CRUNCHER WORLD FACT BK. U.S. HIST. ON CD-ROM LIBRARY OF THE FUTURE	WORD CRUNCHER WORLD FACT BK. U.S. HIST. ON CD-ROM LIBRARY OF THE FUTURE	1990
NEW CD-ROM TITLES AS THEY ARE PUBLISHED!	NEW CD-ROM TITLES AS THEY ARE PUBLISHED!	NEW CD-ROM TITLES AS THEY ARE PUBLISHED!	1991

Figure 1. Reference works in special media

While we all appreciate the fact that word processors and other technological developments make life easier and allow us to access information more efficiently, the technological growth of the past decade has had a greater effect on the impaired population than the non-impaired population. Personal computers allow many to accomplish tasks that make them competitive in school, work and life. Researchers point out that the largest pool of untapped labor resources (those who want to be gainfully employed) is the disabled. Statistics indicate that only 18 percent of the disabled population is employed full time and only 9 percent is employed part time; the rest are unemployed, not because of lack of desire but because people do not understand the capabilities of the disabled. There is no better place to demonstrate ability than in education. Libraries and librarians have the responsibility to provide access to information and demonstrate that the "disabled" and "temporarily-abled"[3] share the same learning environment. The mission statement of most public and academic libraries, like that of The American Library Association, includes a proviso for providing access to information for all, regardless of economic background, color, creed or disability.[4] The following chapters will explain why and how you can adapt equipment you may already have or can purchase for a modest sum.

Acknowledgments

To my friends and colleagues of the Cleveland Public Library and the National Library Service for the Blind and Physically Handicapped Network...thank you for your tolerance, humor, intellectual stimulation...and most of all for always being willing to listen or help.

Appreciation also goes to James M. Mates for engineering many of the charts and figures and to the Cleveland Sight Center for allowing me to take photographs of some of its equipment.

Author's Note

The products included for discussion in this book are representative only. Their inclusion, or the inclusion of vendors over similar products/vendors does not constitute an endorsement by the author. The author was not able to personally test all products and was reliant on product and consumer descriptions. Prices quoted are the approximate retail prices for 1991.

1

Technology and the Disabled—Surveying Your Needs

While the scientific research field has many units which strive to make our world and our lives better, the "adaptive technology" branch with its emphasis on computer adaptions for the disabled has given the disabled a second chance to live competitively in the world. There are many types of disabilities which prevent persons from sitting down and accessing computer information directly (i.e., sitting at a computer and typing information and visually reading the information from the screen, without any added device). Finding the perfect solution to enable all to access information is neither an easy task nor one that is ever finished.

Persons with physical disabilities such as severe arthritis or multiple sclerosis have difficulty inputting information into computers (i.e., operating the keyboard, mouse and other devices that are used to control the computer).[1] These patrons may not possess enough dexterity to handle a diskette or a paper tray. For these persons, alternate methods of inputting information such as voice command, rocker switches or loading trays may be needed.

People with sensory disabilities such as visual impairment experience difficulty getting information from the computer, primarily because the accepted form of information transfer comes from one viewing the monitor screen. For individuals who have difficulty seeing the screen, or who are completely unable to see the screen, alternate display methods such as a large print screen, voice or braille may be required.

People who have language disorders such as aphasia or learning disabilities such as dyslexia may be able to profit from alternate input and output devices, but primarily need assistance in message formulation, perception, and other areas, which are still in great need of research.[2]

There are several ways for individuals with disabilities to use a personal computer. One is by using software specifically developed for the disabled user. This would include programs such as text-to-braille (braille-to-text) translators, talking screen programs, and programs for enlarging print. Special word processing programs are also available, to be used in place of mass-market programs such as WordPerfect or Multi-Mate, which segregate the user and impose limits. The most useful way to use adapted technology is by coupling it with standard information such as that found on CD-ROM discs or online networks; using the technology in this way causes the access door to information to swing open.

This method—modifying the operating system software in the computer—allows the disabled individuals to use the same programs as the nondisabled users. For instance a person with very little dexterity who is unable to use a keyboard may be able to use a Morse-code switch. With a Morse-code translator installed within the operating system, a user can tap three "dashes" on a computer and an "S" will appear where the patron wants it.[3]

These same changes can be made to the operating system to call up braille displays and voice outputs. There are software programs that will translate audible signal beeps into screen flashes.

While these software programs work most of the time they are not foolproof. Professionals using braille translating programs say that "while the software may occasionally mistranslate a braille contraction, they are good and valuable."[4]

Still another method of giving access to all computer functions is the most expensive, but also the most "user friendly" (i.e., it will not interfere with any operation of the computer or the software): hardware adaptions, such as modified or special alternate keyboards, disk drives or displays, which are added to a standard computer configuration.

Some examples of easy "add-ons" for use by the physically disabled include a "micro keyboard" for those who have a limited finger extension or range or a large "expanded keyboard" in place of the standard keyboard for those whose fine motor control is limited. In some cases the standard keyboard may be replaced by an "optical light beam" attached to headband. These keyboard emulations are designed in a manner which enables the standard keyboard to remain connected allowing the disabled and the nondisabled users to share the computer.

While the physically disabled need a way to physically input the information, the blind or visually disabled need some type of output device such as a screen enlarger (which can be as simple as a "screen-sized" magnifier or a large-print software program) or a speech synthesizer which, when coupled with a screen reading program, converts and reads aloud written ASCII text. Some blind users could also use "dynamic braille displays" which allow them to read the screen by feeling small pins raise and lower, emulating braille.

Alternate output and input allows the blind or visually or physically disabled to read everything that the sighted and "physically-abled" person can. The disabled who use a personal computer have called it a variety of affectionate and cogent terms such as "the great equalizer," "an extension of myself," and "my missing parts place."

Unlike most members of society who use the personal computer primarily to do things faster and more efficiently, the disabled use the computer to gain knowledge, job skills and an independent life! These are the same service goals that most of us in libraries hope to reach, so it is perfectly logical for you to set aside budget dollars to include computer adaptions to make your library more accessible to the disabled.

There is much that can be done with existing technology to aid the disabled. One of the most difficult tasks you face will be to decide what to do first; another task will be putting it all together and making it work. The third task will be to keep growing and working as technology grows.

Is There Really a Need for This Special Technology?

Most librarians, when asked to make adjustments to their facilities to better serve the disabled, are quick to say, "but there are no disabled people coming into my library, why should I spend the money to make the library more accessible?" This is indeed a "catch-22"-type question which can best be answered by saying, "if there is nothing in your library why should they come?" Someone must take the initiative, and it should be the person trained to disseminate knowledge.

To determine long-range need, look at the present user group: it is quickly aging. Most acquired disabilities come with age. Figure 1 indicates the projected number of persons 65 years old and older by the year 2000; most will have some type of disability.

Determining the Prevalence of Impairment in Your Community

Blindness and Visual Impairment

Task one requires that your present needs and your anticipated needs be surveyed. Although this sounds like the easiest task (i.e., simply turn it over to your planning and research department), it is not. For instance, most states do not keep blindness statistics, so finding an accurate number of persons currently blind may be next to impossible. Estimating the total number of visually impaired people may be impossible because in its simplest, yet accepted definition, visual impairment is the inability to correct vision (with a glass prescription) in a manner to allow the reading of standard print (10 pt). A person who is visually impaired (rather than being blind) will not appear to have a disability, as he or she will not be using a white cane or guide dog to navigate. Additionally, visually impaired people may not admit they are impaired either because they do not wish to call attention to themselves and wish to remain in the mainstream or they do not feel that society should adjust to them. Visually impaired persons, however, will probably have to use a magnifier to read or hold the material very close to their eyes; they may even avoid read-

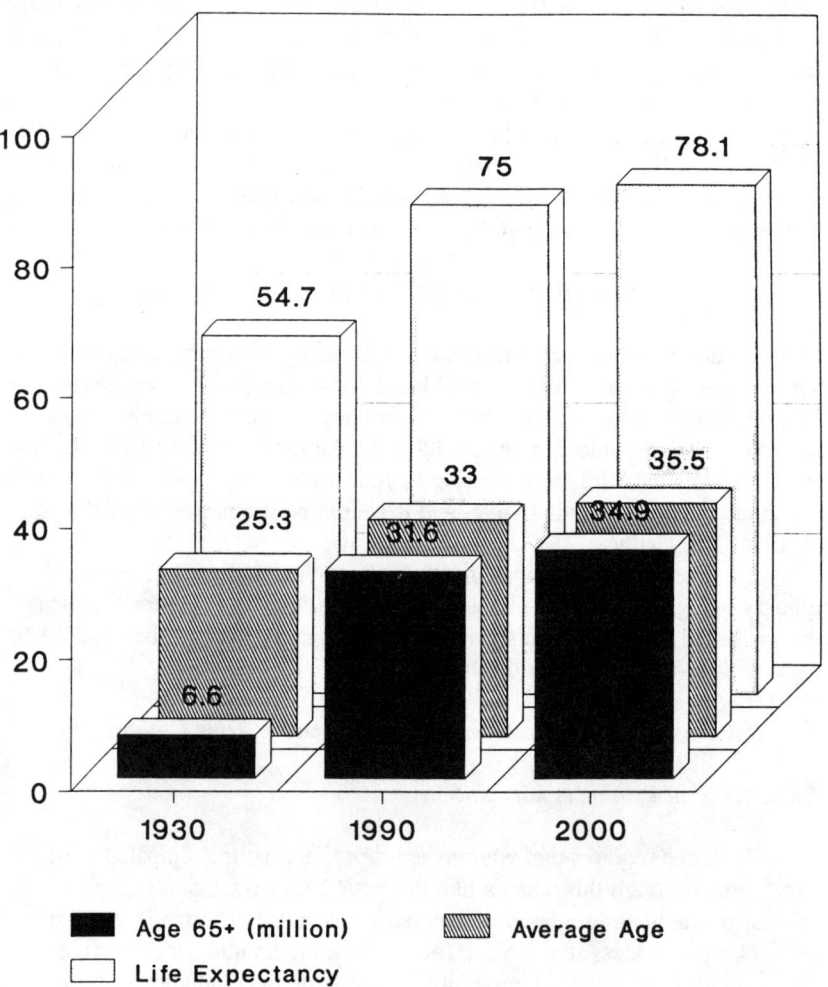

Figure 1. The maturing of the U.S. population. Source: *1988 Statistical Abstract--U.S.*

ing. Nevertheless, there are sources that can be checked and disabilities estimated.

At the present time the highest incidence of acquired visual impairment occurs within the population of 65 years and over. As the population continues to age so will the number of people acquiring some type of visual impairment. Figure 2 indicates the past and present distribution of older Americans

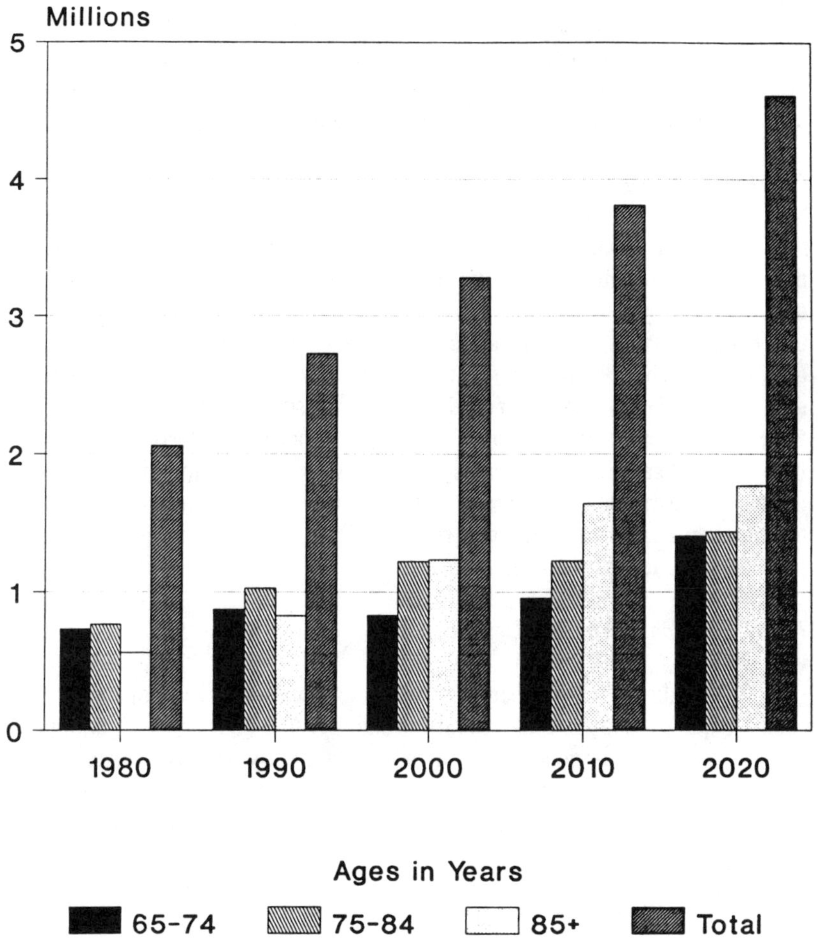

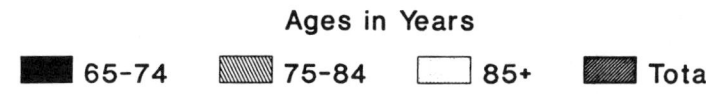

Figure 2. Prevalence of severe visual impairment—United States

with severe visual impairment as well as the estimated population by the year 2020; if all factors remain constant (i.e., no miracle cure for eye diseases such as macular degeneration and no sudden mortality wave), there will be a dramatic growth in the need for devices to aid the impaired. This would imply that if you are in an area that has a dense population of older people, you may anticipate a population growth of visually impaired patrons.

While aging is the major contributor to visual impairment, there are other diseases that cause those afflicted to lose vision to the degree of not being able to read normal print material. Juvenile diabetes is a contributor to acquired blindness in children and young adults. Uncontrolled diabetes also causes temporary or permanent blindness in adults. There are also many viruses such as AIDS whose treatment has visual impairment as a possible side effect. If your community tracks these diseases, you may want to check the incidence of these diseases, as well as other blindness-contributing illnesses.

Physical Impairment

Physical impairment determination in relation to reading impairment is the most difficult number to determine. While we are able to look at the annual statistics provided by the National Library Service, we must keep in mind that these statistics are only indicative of registered patrons (NLS estimates that it is reaching only 5 percent of eligible users) who have indicated that they are physically unable to read a book. Statistics compiled by the Census Bureau, in a report titled, "Labor Force and Other Characteristics of Persons with Work Disabilities," indicates that the number is growing and will continue to grow. Birth defects, disease and trauma lead less often to death than impairment and disability. Figure 3, reflects the number of persons who become physically disabled on an annual basis.

Hearing Impairment and Deafness

Like other statistics, hearing impairment and deafness statistics are not easily acquired. This is due partially to the fact that hearing loss (as opposed to deafness which is genetic) is for most a gradually acquired disability that people do not want to acknowledge. The 1990 Census expects to find three

- 8,000 surviving spinal cord injury each year
- 420,000 surviving brain trauma each year
- 20 million with arthritis
- 1.5 million with neurological disorders
- 17 million with hearing impairment
- 8.2 million with visual impairment
- 70% of population will at some time be so disabled that they cannot climb a flight of stairs

Figure 3. Incidence of disability. Based on a report issued by the U.S. Census Bureau "Labor Force and Other Characteristics of Persons with Work Disabilities, 1981-1986."

million persons over 85 experiencing an appreciative hearing loss, which prevents them from fully participating in "life" activities.[5] Figure 4 indicates the growing number of persons having or developing a hearing impairment since the year 1971.

While the Census does have its problems (e.g., currency in reporting process), it should not be overlooked. And organizations like the National Institutes of Health and the American Foundation for the Blind[6] do keep statistics and are willing to discuss projections with you.

Appendix 1 lists the number of registered readers in all the states and its possessions (this is a combined list of both visually and physically im-

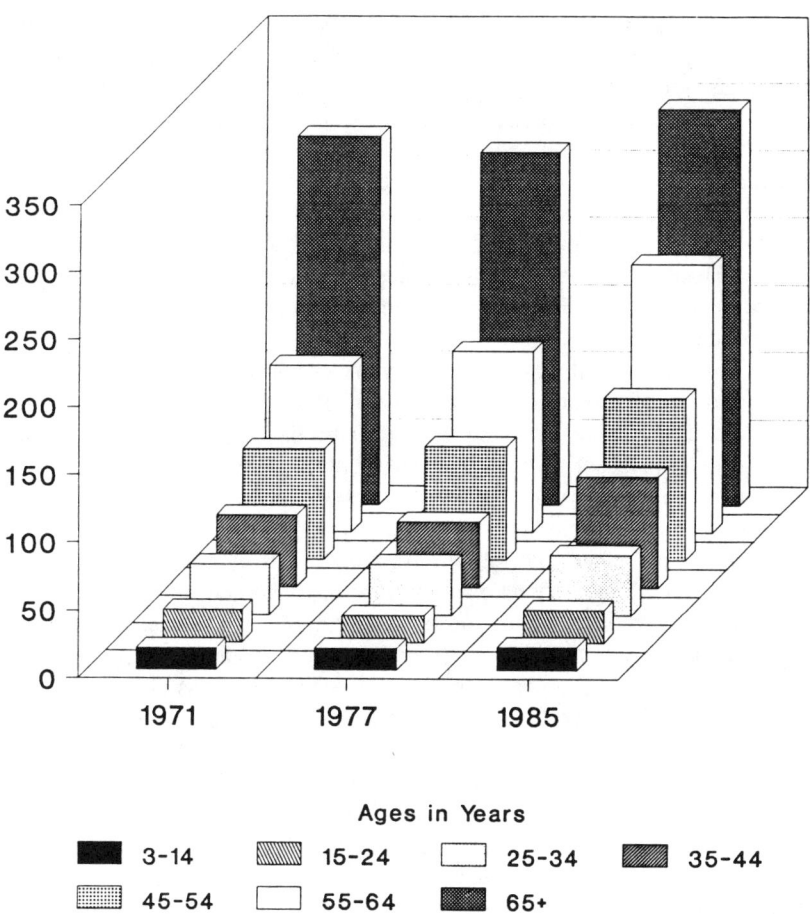

Figure 4. *Persons with impaired hearing per thousand, by age. Source: National Center for Health Statistics*

paired). Since the National Library Service estimates that it is currently reaching only 5 percent of the eligible readers, these figures should be multiplied by the per capita library usage in your community.

After Research—First Steps

When you survey your population you will more than likely determine that visual impairment is the fastest growing group needing library and print access and that the largest proportion of this group will be using large print. Large print is the media which most people turn to first—it simply is one step up from using a magnifier with regular print materials. The person is still able to get reading material either in book or newsprint format. Large print makes readers feel that they are still part of the mainstream. The National Association for the Visually Handicapped estimates that 97 percent of those who will live to 80 will need large-print materials.[7]

When reading large print is no longer possible, people turn to the recorded format. The cassette recorder has never been as popular as it is now. It has grown from being the recording novelty of the mid-seventies to being one of the strongest formats of the nineties. Many commuters are listening to books as they travel to work and others are listening to them as a family experience. All of this listening we are doing makes listening to synthetic speech the next natural step. Grocery stores and banks are preparing us for this type of communication.

The National Library Service Network provides equipment and deposit collections to all libraries requesting them. Patrons tend to have an easier transition time if they are taken through it by their neighborhood librarian. Acquiring this type of technology for your library is as simple as picking up the phone and calling your cooperating Network Library.

If so many people are reading large print and listening to the spoken text, why even bother with braille? As noted, there is a time when reading large print is no longer possible and in some cases was never possible. Braille is actually the preferred media for persons born blind or blinded early in life. More discussion on the "whys" of braille can be found in Chapter 4. Although it is not a "technological notion," deposit collections of braille can be arranged by your network librarian; this paves the way for the advances you are about to make.

In summation, if funds are limited it is suggested that large-print applications be explored first, as they are the easiest and most economical to bring to fruition. This medium is also what most commercial computer personnel will be familiar with—you can go into a local store and purchase a mass-market printer that will give you large print; you cannot do this with any of the other adaptions we will address.

Overall Warning

If you are purchasing a new PC to use with your adaptions or thinking of using one of your current PCs for the adaptions, it is best to talk with the adaptions vendors and ask them what type of PC is best to purchase and what problems to anticipate if you cannot use the type of computer they suggest. The newest and the most expensive is not always the best choice. A perfect example of this occurred when the Cleveland Regional Library decided to upgrade its rapidly aging IBM-XT. Thinking it better to stick with a proven brand, we purchased an IBM PC/386 and thought we could transfer the voice card to the new unit. The card was physically too big for the micro-channel chassis (the PC salesman had told us everything from the old PC could be transferred) and so we had to purchase a new, more expensive card. Had we sought someone knowledgeable in the protocol of adaptive technology we would not have had any problems.

The source list included in this book (Appendix 2), while not inclusive, is made up of companies that: 1) have visually or physically impaired persons on staff, using and refining the actual products; 2) have people who will return your calls (even if they know your problem is not their product's fault but the fault of your PC) and help you work through your crisis.

Keep in mind that the marketplace for products that allow people to use computers has been fragmented and slow to develop. There are about one million people in the U.S. that have some type of disability that prevents them from being able to use a keyboard, and 800 products from almost as many companies.[8] With technology moving as fast as it is, products quickly become obsolete and small companies and developers cannot handle the losses having old stock brings; also, it should be pointed out that disabled individuals do not have a lot of money to spend purchasing, let alone upgrading, their equipment. Since companies in this area come and go with considerable frequency, it is wise to stick with proven products and seek a distributor with sales representatives in your area who can come on site for a product demonstration.

If you are computer literate, or working with a computer-literate person and wish to go it alone, the following rule of thumb should be observed when buying the basic PC: the computer you purchase should have enough expansion slots, memory, speed, and power to run your adaptive equipment as well as your off-the-shelf hardware and software.[9] Lloyd Rasmussen, a colleague employed by the National Library Service and a proficient computer user, once advised me, "If cost is not a factor, get the fastest PC currently available with as many expansion slots open as possible plus an extra serial port (for a braille printer)." His sage advice allowed an IBM-XT to grow beyond what most people thought possible of an XT. While there are some who say a PC with one megabyte is sufficient,[10] it is suggested that, if your budget will allow, you should invest the extra dollars and get two megabytes. Memory-resident programs as well as DOS (version 4.1 and below) gradually eat up the memory and you find yourself having to make bootable disks to save memory and allow the use of some CD-ROM configurations. As we all know, new and exciting innovations are being developed every day which we do not know about until they are introduced and advertised. Since it is inconceivable to know which products you are going to be able to purchase to add on to your system, the extra megabyte gives you room to grow.

2

Large-Print Access

Large print is the easiest and least expensive alternate adaption to make (both for the information giver and the information receiver). We are all familiar with advertising done in several typefaces and are aware that some are easier to read than others. With the information overload we experience every day, I'm sure all will agree that the easiest to read gets read first. Large print will be appreciated not only by the visually impaired user but also by the non-impaired user who would like information that is easier to see and a terminal that is easier to view.

A question that often arises concerning large print is: "What is actually considered large print?" Large print is legally defined as typeface larger than 13.9 pt.[1] The example in Figure 1 illustrates common point sizes used in

> This is an example of 12 pt. print. This typeface is used periodically by printers for popular books, paperbacks and shorter correspondence.
>
> THIS IS AN EXAMPLE OF 14 PT. PRINT. THIS TYPEFACE IS SELDOM SEEN IN MASS MARKET PRINTING, BUT IS THE NORM IN THE LARGE PRINT PUBLISHING OF BOOKS AND MAGAZINES. PERSONS WITH IMPAIRED VISION CAN READ THIS PT. TYPE WITH A CORRECTIVE LENS AND/OR MAGNIFIER.
>
> THIS IS AN EXAMPLE OF 16 PT. PRINT. THIS TYPEFACE IS NEVER SEEN IN MASS MARKET PRINTING AS THIS TYPEFACE REQUIRES 30% MORE PAPER AND WOULD MAKE THE AVERAGE BOOK COSTLY AND CUMBERSOME. IT IS USED BY LARGE PRINT PUBLISHERS AND BY THOSE WISHING TO USE A TYPEFACE WHICH COULD BE EASILY ACCESSED BY THE VISUALLY IMPAIRED.
>
> THIS IS AN EXAMPLE OF 18 PT. PRINT. THIS TYPEFACE IS EASY TO SEE ONE LETTER AT A TIME BUT IS RARELY USED IN THE PRINTING WORLD, AS MOST VISUALLY IMPAIRED USERS FIND IT DIFFICULT TO READ BECAUSE WORDS BECOME TOO SPREAD OUT AS THEY SCAN THE PRINTED PAGE.

Figure 1. Comparative type

printing. Note how much easier it is to read the examples of "large print" than standard print.

There are various adaptions that can be made which give the patron the ability to "interface" with the hardware as well as getting large print output. They cover the gamut of budget allotments and yield various amounts of large print access. If your budget is limited, provide what your budget will allow. Whichever access point is eased will be one less barrier that will have to be overcome.

Keyboards

Viewing the standard keyboard is a problem for the visually impaired computer user. A person accessing the keyboard with some regularity more than likely has memorized the keyboard and does not need to actually see the keys for the input of information. However, for the user who cannot memorize the keyboard layout or the occasional library computer user, there are "large print" keyboard labels called "touchdown keytops" which increase the alpha point size type from 18 pt. to 32 pt. and the numeric point size from 14 pt. to 18 pt. These keytop legends are made of plastic and have an adhesive backing that will stick directly onto the IBM or IBM compatible keys. This is a relatively inexpensive method (under $30) of making the keyboard more accessible to the visually impaired. Figure 2 shows the actual size of the keytops; note how the letter and number fill all the available key area, rather than leave white space.

The one disadvantage to these "peel and stick" keytops is that they can be easily pulled off by someone wishing to pull them off (intentionally), unless you purchase a clear key cap cover for each key, which are sold by Hoolean Corporation and other companies selling standard keyboard accessories. You can purchase the large-print keytops from LS & S Group, Hoolean Corporation and Data Cal Corporation.

A more lasting solution is customized keytops. Hoolean Corporation will make customized keys to your specifications. Ordering customized keys

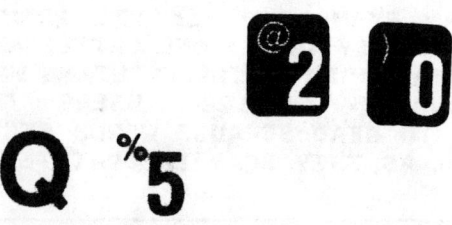

Figure 2. Large-print keytops fill the entire key area, making the keys easier to see for all users.

gives you the opportunity to have commonly used function commands such as "print," "save" and "exit" created as well.

You may also consider a large-print membrane keyboard, which is a flat, pressure-sensitive keyboard with overlays on which large-print keyboard layouts may be used. For more information on the membrane keyboard, please see Chapter 6.

Screen Displays

One can obtain large-print display screens either with hardware adaptions or software adaptions. Software is generally the less expensive approach and tends to inconvenience the non-disabled user the least. The reason for this is that most of the large-print programs are memory resident and must be called up, while physical screen magnifiers are always affixed to the computer.

Software Approach

There are several software packages that will allow the user to enlarge the words on the screen while he or she is using another commercial word processing system such as WordPerfect. All should be installed as memory-resident programs on a hard disk system as this allows for harmonious interaction with other software. Most require at least 40K of free RAM memory and DOS 2.0 or higher. Descriptions of some of the more popular large-print screen programs follow; most have demonstration disks available, which will allow you to determine if the product is easy to use.

ZoomText

Developed by A-1 Squared, ZoomText will enlarge text from 2x (twice normal width and twice normal height) to 8x. There are three built-in fonts which vary in character thickness (from thick to thin) and also possess variable inter-character spacing (helpful for both the user who can see bold characters easily and for the user who is bothered by the spacing that is created with bolder type). The program is menu-driven (see Figure 3) and has many features such as "scrolling" which allow you to magnify and read any portion of the screen at any time. The scrolling feature also allows you to vary the speed by which the words float by. Viewing allows you to see the magnified text in its relation to the full screen of text. There are also "zoom" features (left, right, top, bottom) which will display the normal text and the magnified text at the same time; this is particularly helpful if the user has a greater field of vision in one direction over another. Having the normal text displayed allows the user to have a sense of placement within the working document, as the

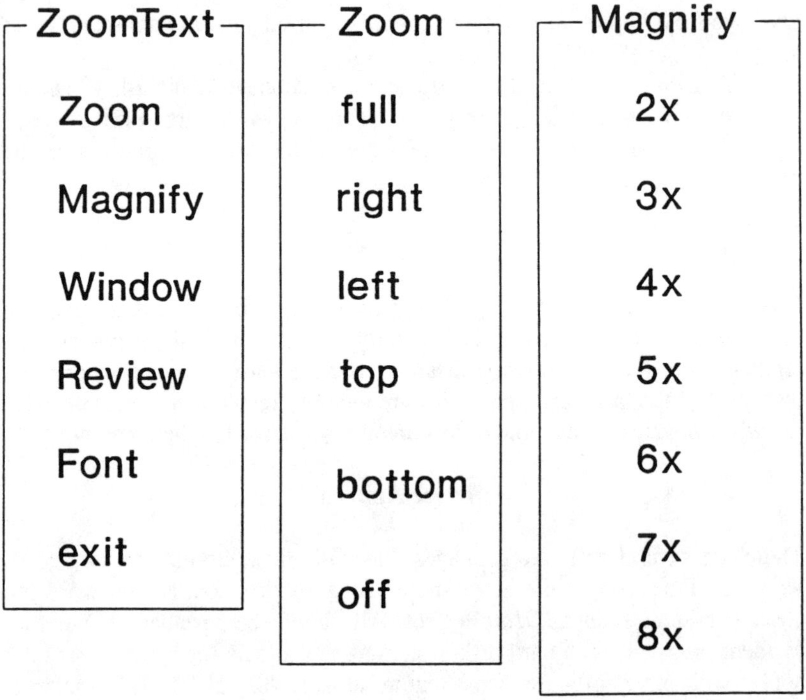

ZoomText	Zoom	Magnify
Zoom	full	2x
Magnify	right	3x
Window	left	4x
Review	top	5x
Font	bottom	6x
exit	off	7x
		8x

Figure 3. ZoomText *has a menu system which allows the user easy access to the large-print screen program.*

magnified screen is only displaying a few words or letters at a time. Another feature worth noting is "reverse video," which causes the background and the letters to reverse for the times when it may be easier to see, for example, blue on yellow instead of yellow on blue.

The program is user-friendly, easy to learn and provides even a novice with clear, easy-to-read enlarged screen characters within a few minutes. The program is approximately $500 and is available from A-1 Squared and its various distributors.

InFocus

InFocus was developed by the same group that developed ZoomText and has most of the same features, the exception being that it has only one font—the 2x magnification. You do have your choice of 2x width, height and twice normal size and height (a good viewing size). It allows the user to access all of the other features of ZoomText. This product is priced extremely economically for the output it gives ($150). It has the same pull-down menus as ZoomText, which make learning easy. It is available from A-1 Squared and its representatives, such as LS & S Group.

PC Lens

PC Lens was designed for an IBM PC, XT, AT or compatibles. This software program requires DOS 3.10 or greater and allows users to magnify the screen 5x to 11x to 20x the standard screen letter size. All four sizes contain the entire 255 IBM PC characters. PC Lens has a dual tracking feature which insures normal software interaction. This program works with a monochrome screen, unless a separate color graphics card is purchased. PC Lens is manufactured by ARTS Computer Products and retails for $500.

Deluxe LP-DOS

Deluxe LP-DOS will enlarge the screen display up to 20x magnification (using a menu similar to the ZoomText menu). The main element of this package, LP-DOS, makes programs such as WordPerfect and Lotus 1-2-3 easy to read for the visually impaired. Its secondary program, "El-Picasso," magnifies graphics and charts which greatly enhances its usage, especially in settings which require the user to refer to illustrations. Like most large-print programs, LP-DOS allows the user access to commercial instructional software packages (such as typing tutors) as well as recreational packages, such as flight simulators. Deluxe LP-DOS was developed by VisionWare and is designed to work with IBM PC, XT, AT, PS/2, laptops and compatibles equipped with EGA, CGA or VGA display adapters. The program also has a built-in feature that acknowledges that IBM clones may have differences which cause the screen to "jitter" in scanning modes and allows the user to "track" the display until the reading is stable. LP-DOS is priced at $500 and is available from Optelec and various representatives, such as Celexx Corp.

Soft Vista

Developed and supported by TeleSensory Products (TSI), the Soft Vista program is unique in that it has its own mouse. Soft Vista's mouse attaches directly to the circuit board and allows the user to stretch an image taller, wider and both, simply by pressing one of the three buttons on the mouse, thus eliminating the need of menus for font choice, enlarging features or contrast features. This program, however, will not enlarge graphics or give you the presentation view feature that other programs do. Soft Vista will work on an IBM PC (or clone), including the micro-channel model. The program is supported by TSI and has a toll-free customer support service. Most of the prod-

16 *Library Technology for Visually and Physically Impaired Patrons*

uct developers and support personnel are users of the products they sell and advise you from the user's knowledge base rather than a salesperson's point of view. This product runs little chance of interfering with application programs because of the fact that the mouse directs its own cursor about the screen allowing free and random screen access. This product is available from TSI and representatives throughout the country for approximately $2,500.

Artic Focus

Artic Focus is a new addition (Spring 1991) to the large-print software field. It was created by Artic Technologies, a respected leader in adaptive technology. The menu operation allows one to quickly enlarge screen text from 1-10x's and offers simple but solidly formed letters (see Figure 4). It works well with commercial packages such as WordPerfect and dBase. As an added plus, it will also work synchronously with Artic Visions (which it also produces), one of the most popular speech screen access packages available.

SIZE	COLOR
1X FONT	
2X FONT	
3X FONT	
4X FONT	
6X FONT	
8X FONT	
10X FONT	

Figure 4. *Artic Focus gives user menus to make choosing attributes easier.*

This large-print adapter will work with all versions of the IBM PC (or compatible) and allows the reader to bypass unwanted screen updating and text presentation by jumping or "snapping" directly to the desired point (Snap-Tool feature).

For ease in using the program Artic Technologies has added a hardware device called "Gizmo," which gives the user all of the aforementioned capabilities without having to use the keyboard, which means the system can be accessed at all times. The Gizmo does cost extra but allows the occasional user to learn the system faster and the advanced user to develop macros to gain even quicker output. The technical staff is top-notch and publishes a free, quarterly newsletter, *Visions,* with helpful usage hints about its products.

Panorama and Powerama

A newcomer to the large print scene in the United States (although widely known in Canada) is the Panorama Large Print Program, developed and distributed by Syntha-Voice Computers of Hamilton, Ontario. This package offers three letter thicknesses and up to 10x magnification fonts. It promises smooth movement without the screen "jitters" and possesses an infinite color palate, as well as numerous shades of black. It is easy to move about the screen by simply using the page up and page down command. It works well with word processing programs and has the ability to use calculator programs as well. Powerama includes all the features of Panorama but adds the synthetic voice screen review. These programs work with an IBM and require 35K RAM.

Reminders

We have just discussed a few of the many large-print display screen software packages available (see Figure 5). There are other programs in the software arena including public domain software that may adequately do the job for your user. Ask for a demonstration disk before purchasing, as most of the products discussed here have them available.

The one thing to keep in mind with all of these packages is that the presentation of the large print will be only as good as the monitor on which it is being displayed. Any one of these translators' screen-displays will look better and be easier to read on a quality screen with higher resolution than on a lower-resolution monitor.

Remember, too, that the company which provides a toll-free customer support line staffed by assistants who actually know how to use the program can save you a lot of frustration and many long-distance phone bills.

	Magnification range	Able to vary letter thickness	Able to vary letter spacing	Menu driven	Top/bottom magnification	Left/right magnification	Screen scan control	Normal screen view	RAM required	Cost	Other
Artic Focus	1.5x-10x	NO	NO	YES	YES	YES	YES	YES	100K	$550-795	Snap tool
InFocus	2x	YES	NO	YES	NO	NO	YES	YES	50K	$150	
PC Lens	5x,11x,20x	NO	YES	NO	YES	YES	YES	YES	97K	$500	Dual tracking
DeLuxe LP-DOS	2x-20x	YES	YES	YES	YES	YES	YES	YES	75-85K	$500	Graphics pkg
Soft Vista	3x-16x	YES	YES	has own	YES	YES	YES	NO	20-60K	$2500	Has own control
ZoomText	2x-8x	YES	YES	YES	YES	YES	YES	YES	40K	$500	Reverse video
Panorama	2x-10x	YES	YES	NO	YES	YES	YES	YES	35K	$600	Infinite color palate

Figure 5. Large-print software programs

Hardware

There are two hardware approaches to large print and they are vastly different. One approach (accessory lens) is a passive device and requires little technical skill to install or use. The lens will only enlarge material that is being displayed on the video display terminal or personal computer monitor. This method, while limited, is the least costly route.

The other (CCTV) is a stand-alone unit which will enlarge any print reading material (as well as photographs) which is placed on the gliding platform which is mounted beneath a solid-state CCD camera. There are controls which allow the user to adjust the magnification, brightness, and contrast of the image which is projected onto the monitor. Some CCTVs also have the capability of interfacing with a computer screen to yield the viewer magnification capabilities of up to 80x for screen displays. This method, while more costly, is flexible and conducive to growth.

Accessory Lens—COMPU-LENZ

This is the only CRT magnification lens widely available in the marketplace. The COMPU-LENZ uses a unique patented system to increase the character size up to 4x (depending on the size of the screen) as well as filter out glare and reflection. The increase in character size is due to the high-powered Fresnel lens. This lens is diamond cut in a series of concentric grooves etched into a plastic material (polymethylmetacrylate) and spaced a few thousandths of an inch apart. Although the screen is curved it appears absolutely flat. It is a neutral gray filter which makes each character stand out clearly from the background. If you are proficient in the use of DOS or have a word processing program that allows you to change the environment, this filter offers a chance to experiment with various shades.

COMPU-LENZ is as easy to install as a commercial screen filter—simply mount it with velcro to the monitor. It is priced at $200; however, for a nominal amount the manufacturer also offers a more permanent mount called a "swivel mount." This device has arms, slides under the monitor and allows the installer to slide COMPU-LENZ into the support clips (see Figure 6). This method does away with the slippage that is so common with velcro attachments. COMPU-LENZ is widely available from LS & S, VIS-AIDS, Ann Morris and other distributors of products for the visually impaired.

If considering this type of large-print adaption remember that while this is the easiest (i.e., does not require installer to have any computer installation knowledge) and most economical approach to large-print screen display, there are other considerations as well: 1) it is essentially permanent which means that all users of the personal computer you put it on will be forced to

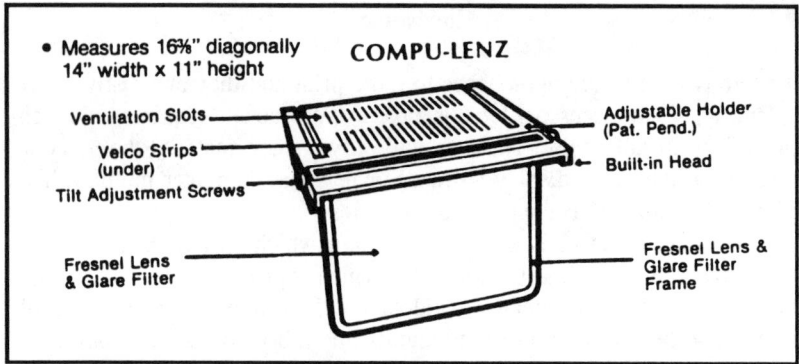

Figure 6. The COMPU-LENZ slips on the monitor as easily as an anti-glare screen.

use the magnification as well (this could also be seen as an advantage as students who are spending hours in front of the screen may actually prefer the larger print to reduce eye strain); 2) 4x is the maximum magnification power and it is a fixed magnification (unlike the software approach); and 3) although it is a high-quality plastic the lens is still plastic, which has a tendency to scratch easily and does not possess the clarity of glass.

CCTV Systems

While they are more expensive than software for computers or a magnifier for a terminal screen, Closed Circuit Televisions and or Displays (CCTVs or CCDs) can turn your entire print library into a large-print library for anyone with as little as 1 percent of normal vision. They can also aid the visually impaired patrons who simply want to read their correspondence, view snapshots of their grandchildren or read the daily newspaper, and they have the capability to interface with and enlarge computer screens. There also are several systems which can enlarge material onto a projection screen up to 80x's.

The basic system works much like a microfiche reader. Printed items are placed on a gliding platform mounted beneath a camera lens. Controls adjust the magnification, brightness and contrast of the image that is projected to the monitor above. These systems will also allow the user wishing to write checks or letters to view documents as they are being composed by placing writing material on the platform and writing. The price range varies with the display unit size and by added features such as zoom lenses or color monitors. Most units come with a color camera which allows shade variations (this feature is also available for black and white monitors). With one exception, the non-portable models will take up at least two square feet of space. They will fit in a study carrel, leaving plenty of space for a computer. The most widely known systems are made by TeleSensory Products, Optelec, Big Vue and Seeing Technologies. Figure 7 is representative of all the CCTVs capable of PC interface.

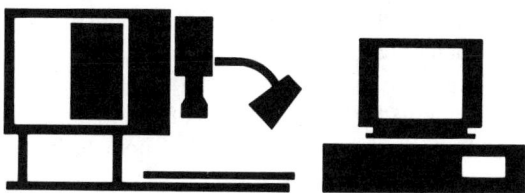

Figure 7. User can view the camera image and the computer screen simultaneously. Diagram courtesy Optelec.

TeleSensory Products. TeleSensory Products (TSI) has a complete line of CCTVs. The most versatile model for the dollar is Vantage ($2,500). Vantage possesses one feature that sets it apart from other CCTVs and that is its "floating monitor," which raises and lowers itself over the object it's magnifying—allowing for large volumes to be placed beneath it. There is also a solid-state camera which actually monitors what it is focusing on and projects it onto the screen. Vantage CCD's 14-inch monitor can actually enlarge the image up to 45x. A more elite model, the Voyager XL, magnifies the print up to 60x on a 19-inch black and white monitor. Common features of all of the CCTVs from TeleSensory include many of the standards found in the large-print software programs, i.e., image reversal, brightness control, windowing (blocking out areas of the display), tilt screen and two camera screens (this allows one to read and write on the same platform by adjusting each camera to proper projection height). All of these controls are adjusted with dials on the front of the machine.

TSI also has an adaptive device called Lynx which is able to link one of its CCTVs to a personal computer. By linking the PC to the CCTV the entire library opens up to the visually impaired user. The patron is now able to read any book in the library (as well as have a place to read and write his/her personal correspondence), use the online catalog (if available through the PC) or search any CD-ROM title that the library owns. TSI offers a toll-free assistance line and product representatives are strategically assigned throughout the country. The products are made in the United States and Ireland and carry a one-year warranty, with the option to purchase extended warranty. TSI is also willing to ship "loaner" machines via next day delivery (the customer pays the cost) if a machine is in transit to it for repair. While the customer is welcome to purchase products directly from TSI, there is a network of representatives throughout the country who are willling to demonstrate the products.

Optelec. Optelec is also a respected leader in the production of CCTVs. Its units come with a 19" high-resolution monitor and high-quality camera lens. Depending on the model they will enlarge documents from 8x to 60x magnification. The basic model (FDR23) will magnify items placed on its platform up to 45x and project the material onto a black and white (or reversed) screen; this unit is self contained, that is, the camera is attached to the monitor which is mounted over the viewing platform.

Optelec also has two models that interface easily with a PC: the FDR23C and the Twenty/20. The FDR23C offers features such as split-screen viewing and will interface with LP-DOS. This interface ability means that the impaired user can look at the magnified PC screen and further enlarge it on the CCTV. The twenty/20 model is worth considering if space is a factor, as this model uses only 14 square inches of desk space yet has the same features found on the FDR models (i.e., split screen, swivel and tilt). Optelec offers a motorized zoom/focus feature and a motorized table as individual options. All of Optelec's products are priced competitively (approximately $2,500, depending on features) and carry a two-year warranty with a guaranteed response time. Although Optelec itself does not maintain a toll-free number, it has both national and international customer support. Its representatives are willing to return customer's phone calls and help match the potential client with the right product.

SeeTec. Seeing Technologies, the manufacturer of SeeTec systems, believes "a world full of color should be viewed in color" which means that its best sellers all have high-resolution color cameras. Because of this company's dedication to producing a better product for the disabled, it received the 1990 Minnesota Governor's Award for "achievement in the area of technology-related assistance for individuals with disabilities."

Its top-of-the-line model, the STC 20, has a 20" color monitor with 450 lines of resolution and will enlarge images placed on its platform up to 60x. Its top-of-the-line black and white monitor has 700 lines of resolution and has the reverse background feature found in many of the large-print programs. All of SeeTec's magnification devices are able to interface with a VHS playback unit and three of its CCTV models are capable of interfacing with a PC. All of Seeing Technologies' units have a one-year guarantee, carry a price tag of $2,100-$2,500 (depending on model) and have area service representatives ready to answer questions concerning its products. The manufacturer does not have a toll-free number, but does accept collect calls (it advertises this aspect of its service quite prominently). Its complete line is also available through L S & S Group.

	Maximum magnification	Monitor size	Monitor type (BW/C)	Adjustable platform	Computer interface	Warranty	Cost
TeleSensory	45-60x	14-19"	YES/NO	YES	YES	1 yr	$2500
Optelec	45-60x	14-19"	YES/NO	NO	YES	2 yr	$2500
SeeTec	60x	20"	YES/YES	NO	YES	1 yr	$2500
Big Vue	60x	13-19"	YES/YES	NO	YES	18 mo	$2900

Figure 8. *CCTVs.*

Big Vue. Big Vue is a line of CCTVs made expressly for LS & S Group, a mail order company catering to the needs of the visually impaired. The seven models with various features are similar to models previously mentioned. All of these models carry an 18-month warranty and all but its budget model will magnify up to 60x. Big Vue's color monitor model, 229-BVC20, will magnify any item placed on its platform (which can be rotated 360 degrees) but does not offer split-screen viewing. Big Vue's color monitor offers the option of black-and-white viewing as well as reverse viewing. Big Vue model 229-BV19SCT-2A offers the same features as the BVC20 on a 19" black-and-white screen but adds the features of split-screen viewing and a "zoom" camera. Big Vue's model 229-BV13 is the bargain of the line. The monitor is an industrial type 13" black-and-white model which will magnify books or any type of reading material up to 45x, but does not have any features such as split-screen viewing or zoom camera viewing. While this model will not interface with a PC, it is lightweight and can be moved about the facility if needed. LS & S maintains a toll-free help line with technicians ready to advise you of the best piece of equipment for your needs.

* * *

The CCTVs or CCDs were one of the first technological success stories. Their strongest point is that they are easy to use and do not tend to intimidate the older patron. They can be used for reading items other than books, which again is a plus for the older patron seeking independent living (i.e., writing checks, reading letters and bills). And the new generation of units will interface with computers, virtually "re-opening" the information world to the visually impaired. We have discussed only some of the more prominent CCTVs and CCDs; there are others available for less money which have lesser magnifications and lower-resolution monitors. Used units of the earliest models are probably available also. If these are all your budget will allow do not hesitate to purchase one until you can afford something better; they will at least allow some users more access.

Large-Print Hardcopy (Output)

Printing materials in large print is an option to which you may unknowingly have access. Many printers possess the ability to generate a multitude of font sizes simply by selecting the typeface you want directly on the printer.

While the dot-matrix printers allow you to stretch the letters to large type, these letters become distorted and thin as they are stretched. It is advisable to purchase a laser printer with the ability to select fonts and typefaces. Laser printers yield clean, non-distorted lines; the letters are perfectly formed and perfectly spaced. The amount of white space around each letter is important, which is why choosing a large print font with a default pitch with this space is equally important.

When selecting a font be sure to search for one which is bold, such as Hewlett Packard's "Presentor Bold" font which has the ability to adjust from 14 pt. type to 18 pt., and also to render landscape printing and portrait printing. The latter is important if you will be interfacing with and printing from a CD-ROM since many of the reference materials do not allow you to adjust the line spacing. Figure 9 demonstrates three typefaces using large-print

---

THIS IS AN EXAMPLE OF 16 PT. TYPE--1,2,3...

Fig. a

Figure A is a sample of Geneva style; letters are not dense enough, making it difficult to identify several letters.

THIS IS AN EXAMPLE OF 16 PT. TYPE--1,2,3...

Fig. b

Figure B is a sample of Helvetica style; letters are strong and letters have white space around them.

THIS IS AN EXAMPLE OF 16 PT. TYPE--1,2,3...

Fig. c

Figure C is a sample of Helvetica Inserat Roman; letters are spaced too closely making it difficult to distinguish individual letters.

Figure 9. Font style should also be a consideration.

fonts. Figure B is the easiest to read, yet all are 16 pt. typeface. Embellished lettering makes it more difficult to focus on the letter's actual structure. Remember to choose a font without serifs. Also, keep in mind that a font whose letter thicknesses vary is not a good choice. The basic bold stroke is best.

If you are purchasing a large-print font for public usage consider "borrowing" it for the library's correspondence. If your system allows notation fields, a reminder that Mrs. Jones would appreciate notices in large print would prompt you to send her a large-print overdue notice; if it's an automatic notices system, perhaps a flag can be placed on large-print records, which would separate them from the masses and allow you to send them out individually.

3

Braille Access

"The percentage of braille users is so low, in fact only 5 percent of the blind read braille [so the argument goes], why even bother with braille?" The arguments go on to say that "recordings and speech outputs are cheaper than braille and save storage space."[1] The reading of and access to braille is, was and will be a continued source of argument within the blind community. The blind's two most vocal organizations, The National Federation of the Blind (NFB) and the American Congress of the Blind (ACB), have made an effort to reestablish the teaching of braille in mainstream learning environments.[2] These groups also sponsor annual braille reading and writing contests. Braille readers will request braille if it is available and prefer it for a number of reasons, which were summed up by Harvey Laurer, Technology Transfer Specialist, Hines VA Hospital, Hines, Ill.[3] (and confirmed in testimonials by braille readers):

1. Braille leaves the ears free. This facilitates activities like oral reading, lecturing from notes and participating in study groups.
2. Hardcopy braille requires no machines to read it. As with print, it requires only the human body. Braille, like print, can also be read on displays analogous to video terminals. Brailling, like writing, can also be done a variety of ways: by hand, with slate and stylus, by a Perkins brailler (similar to but not a typewriter), a thermoform printing press, a braille printer or a computer terminal (either laptop or desktop).
3. Because braille is usually written on paper information can be filed and retrieved easily as opposed to notes which are recorded. Many impaired computer users do not own a computer and rely on computer access centers, thus information on diskette will not help.
4. Braille is preferred for non-textual tasks. Most computer programmers who use braille prefer reading machine code in braille. Music, math and graphs can nearly always be more directly rendered in braille. Braille is a written code designed

as an exact transcription of the alpha-numeric code which appears as printed characters, which makes the reader aware of exact spellings of new words and phrases.
5. When it comes to creativity, braille is the medium of choice for many. These braille users maintain that they "think best" in braille and compose naturally in braille. They, like the majority of the sighted population, prefer to write their words and sentences rather than dictate them.
6. Hearing-impaired persons have difficulty understanding synthetic speech and prefer their information in braille.
7. Although the deaf-blind make up less than 1 percent of the population, their only media for reading is braille.

As an information giver, it is difficult to imagine that one would turn away potential patrons in their quest for information because they are a different color or creed, but in most instances you are turning away potential readers because they cannot physically read print and require braille to access information and learn. Why would anyone deny a woman like the late Helen Keller access to information, simply because she was (not by choice) a part of the smallest minority? Although Ms. Keller a member of a small minority during her life, her written passages such as "All Sight Is Of The Soul" and "Give Me Wings and Let Me Fly," originally done in braille, have been an inspiration to many a sighted person.

Braille production never ceases to impress the sighted non-user. The raised dots which form distinct cells appear as difficult to read as the Dead Sea scrolls. Likewise, the task of translating print to braille seems formidable as well as expensive.

The thoughts that translating print to braille and giving braille access to computer screens are expensive and formidable are simply fallacies. Like large-print alternate access, braille access is attainable at various budget levels and offers the user limited or complete access to information.

Keyboards/Keytops

The most simplistic keyboard modification which can be done is to identify the home row on a standard keyboard. This procedure can be done in under five minutes and for under five dollars! The process simply involves peeling off adhesive backed key covers which have a raised dot on them and placing them on the home-row keys of your keyboard. This will help the blind patron to know exactly where to place his or her fingers to begin typing in standard print and serves as ongoing orientation. This home-row orientation set is available from L S & S, Hoolean and ComputAbility.

A new product which just entered the marketplace is a complete set of adhesive braille keytops—Braille KeyTop Kit. Like the home-row orientation raised dot toppers, these braille identifiers are easy to install and inexpensive. The KeyTops are clear and will not obscure the letter of the key it is being placed over. The kit provides the braille user with the same alpha-numeric and punctuation prompts that sighted people have when using a standard keyboard. This item is priced at $15.00 and is available from Data Cal.

Both of these minor keyboard modifications allow the blind user to refer to the keyboard as most sighted people do. While keyboards can be memorized (and often are), it is reassuring to peek at the keys to be sure you are on target. Adding either the home-row dots or the complete set of braille keytops will allow the user a more confident access. It is possible to place this overlay over the large-print keytops if a "patient" hand is used.

Screen Access—Paperless Braille Displays

Although it would be ideal to have raised dots on the computer screen, the braille user can now read braille print on a screen with the help of a braille screen reader. Braille screen readers allow the user to read the display screen one line at a time via a braille display unit which has solenoids (i.e., pins—see Figure 1) that raise and lower to form the corresponding braille cell and usually two extra cursor locator solenoids to indicate to the user where the cursor is in relation to what is currently being read. These braille screen readers are usually used in conjunction with a normal keyboard. These units are called "paperless braillers" (also referred to as softcopy, linear and refreshable braille[4]) and provide the blind user with a "movable braille window on the world."[5]

These units, priced around $4,000, are highly sophisticated. A typical paperless braille unit will work with a resident software program to instantly translate any commercial software package or online message that appears on the video display. This paperless braille display allows the same access to information from technical accessories such as CD-ROM as well as the ability to access an online database and use any off-the-shelf software package a sighted person would.

It allows the person to skim the text and read (and print if applicable) only the text they want rather than printing or listening to the entire article (it is difficult to "speed-listen" to synthetic speech, but not difficult to speed-read braille, since it is formatted the same as standard text). Most of the paperless braille displays work in conjunction with a regular keyboard and are compatible with most personal computers. Input to the computer is made with a standard keyboard by typing in standard alpha-numeric codes; output is displayed in both alphanumeric codes and in braille. There are several on the market today.

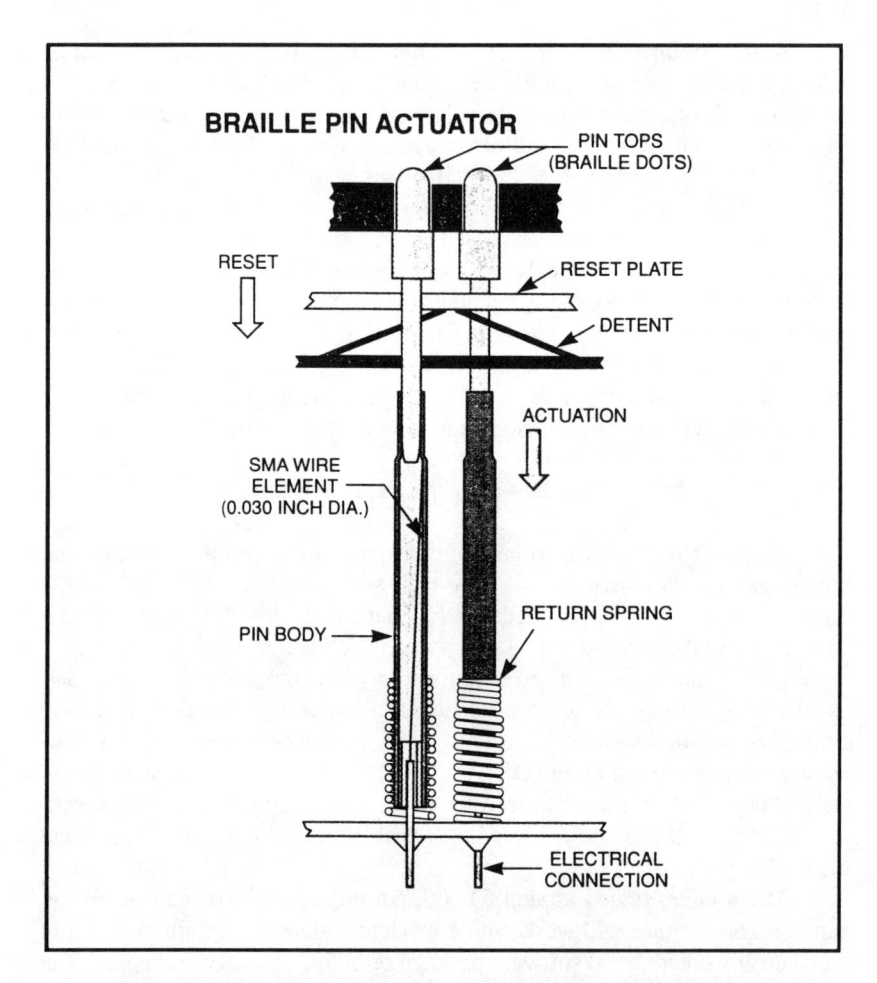

30 *Library Technology for Visually and Physically Impaired Patrons*

Figure 1. There are 32 actuators like this one packed into a small module; five modules form a 20-character line of braille. Source: Lyle McCarty, "Special Alloy Is Key to Braille Display," Design News *29, no.1 (Feb.12, 1990).*

Navigator

Navigator, developed and distributed by TeleSensory Products, Inc. (TSI), is probably the most popular of these paperless braille systems. The actual unit was designed for "unknown" future expansion, which means that the Navigator will currently work with any MS-DOS–based personal desktop computer being sold today as well as several laptop models (Toshiba and Toshiba clones) and will adapt to new PC designs should the user have to upgrade computers (it has extra unused ports).

The Navigator slips under a standard keyboard (it has mounting brackets for laptops) and interfaces with the computer using a RS-232C serial port. You must use one of the two software packages that come with the Navigator to make it of any use, as the software is what actually does the translating and commands the correct solenoid combination to raise and lower when the keys on the keyboard are pressed or the cursor moved. The unit will also signal the user if any screen messages appear (such as error messages) even if they are not working in that sector.

The Gateway software program is what will generally be used as it allows for items such as automatic cursor tracking, high-speed screen searching, movement to a particular line on the screen, a comprehensive screen review and the ability to read windows or columns. This last capability makes access to technical documents easier for the braille user. The one thing it cannot do is translate graphics even if they are bit-mapped.

TSI basically has two models of Navigator which differ dramatically in size and amount of braille displayed (translated). One model is capable of displaying 20 or 40 cells at a time; the other can display 80 cells at a time. The 20- or 40-cell model is quite a bit lighter and is the choice if portability is a concern. If portability or cost are not concerns, the model which displays 80 cells at a time is the model of choice, as it literally doubles the amount of text in braille which can be scanned. While the 80-cell unit is heavier, its dimensions are approximately the same as the 20/40-cell unit.

Octobraille 84

Octobraille 84 is marketed by HumanWare, a company whose "vision and purpose is to help people achieve their potential by providing humanware...the link between technology and people." The Octobraille 84 is easy to install—simply slip it under a standard keyboard and the user has immediate access, in braille, to anything that is displayed on the computer screen. Octobraille, as its name insinuates, yields the user an 80-character, 8-dot display. This hardware unit will allow the highly skilled braille user to program many adaptions and character sets to allow him or her to read the screen quickly.

ALVA

ALVA, also marketed by HumanWare, offers the braille user an 83-cell piezoelectric braille display which uses the three extra dots to serve as reference points so the user knows exactly where he or she is all the time (see Figure 2). The unit not only tells the user where the cursor is but also will relay which screen attributes are active. HumanWare's big selling point for ALVA is that its 80-cell display aligns exactly to the 80 columns of the display

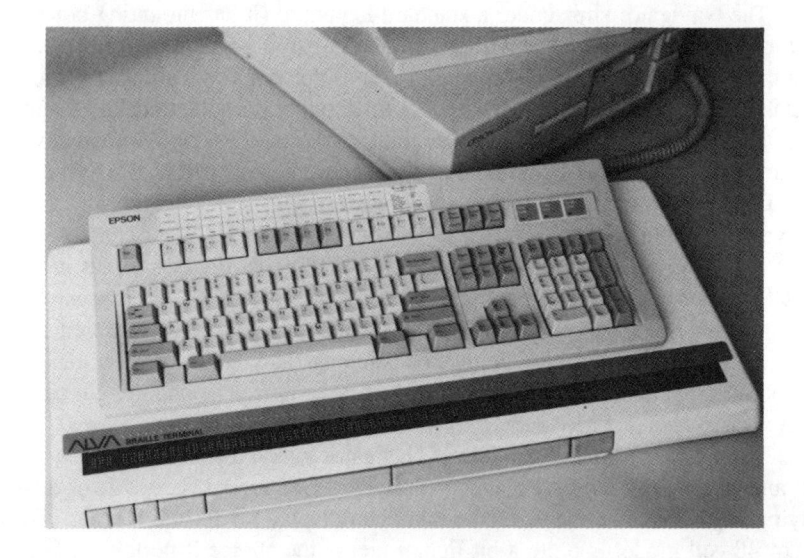

Figure 2. Alva Braille Terminal. There are braille cells that raise and lower translating conventional screen print into braille, which the braille user reads with his/her fingertips. Photo courtesy of HumanWare.

screen, making a highly formatted screen easier to read. It allows the user to see the screen at one time without having to move the cursor to explore the rest of the screen. The unit, priced at approximately $5,000, is available from HumanWare and its representatives nationwide.

Braille n' Speak

While not a true paperless braille unit, quite a few braille users, as well as a training instructor, have told me that I would be remiss if I did not include in this discussion Braille n' Speak, a tremendous bargain. A product of Blazie Engineering (see Figure 3), this unit is priced around $1,000 and interfaces with a computer and enables the user to go online. It also acts as a standalone unit for note-taking (it has only braille entry keys). It is small (8"x4"x1") and lightweight (one pound) yet has the capacity of storing up to 200 pages of braille and has a speech synthesizer installed which is capable of reading the stored braille text aloud. The user would have to use the synthesizer to weed out any unwanted information from storage, but the information would be ready to print in braille, as the unit stores information in Grade II braille. Information can also be formatted in braille and printed in standard print (a special portable printer is even available for this purpose)

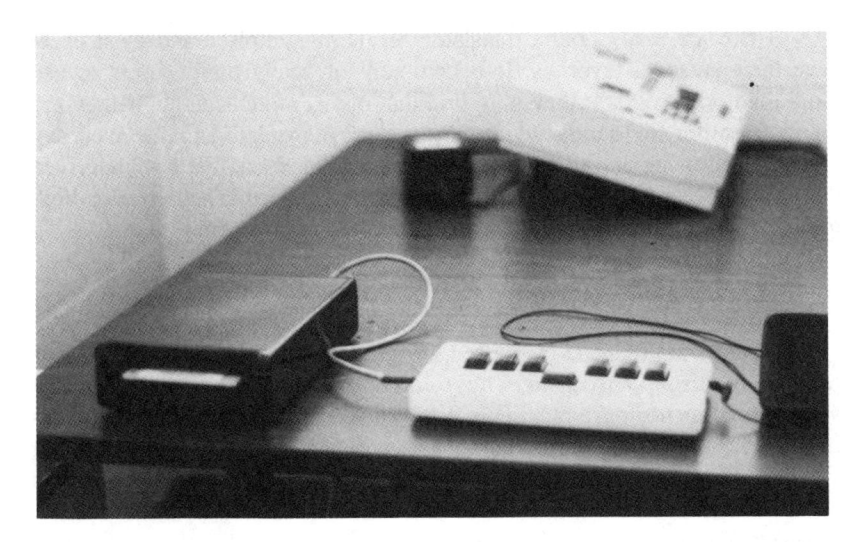

Figure 3. Braille n' Speak uses a minimum amount of desk space, yet can function as a display monitor as well as give the user access to networks.

for instructors or sighted friends. This product is available from E.M. VITU, Inc. and L S & S Group.

Braille Translators: Software for Braille Output from Print

Software braille translators are amazingly accurate, relatively inexpensive (most sell for approximately $500) and are easy to use. They allow any type of information stored as ASCII on the hard disk to be translated within minutes to braille. While it is desirable to have some type of braille printer, the braille translator allows the patron to transfer information in braille code (i.e., encyclopedia articles, prescription information) to a diskette which can be printed when he or she can access a braille printer (either at a school, special needs computer center or a friend's house).

Most of the software programs are easy to use and offer the user print to Grade II braille and Grade II braille to print translations. Since these translators are not foolproof (due to the contextual rules variations in the rules for grade II braille), most of the programs also offer the opportunity to correct mistakes once noticed, so the translator will not make them again (this process is similar to adding a commonly used proper name to your word processor's dictionary so it will not indicate that the word is misspelled every time you use it).

There are many braille translators in the marketplace and most users have their personal favorites. It is common for heavy braille users to use more than one program; they may find that one is more accurate if they are doing scientific translating while they prefer another product for everyday use. The following are among the more popular products that have survived through the years and are in constant updating modes. They receive high marks even from non-users who have occasion to read the translations.

Hotdots Version 3.0

Hotdots is produced by Raised Dots Computing, a small company located in Madison, Wisconsin, whose corporate goal is to help people with visual impairments make maximum use of their computers. Hotdots is an extremely easy-to-use menu-driven software package and with the release of version 3.0 can be used as a batch file operation.

Once the user decides to access Hotdots he or she is given the options menu (see Figure 4).

```
                    Please enter one of the following options:

          _ 1. Import file from word processor (or generic ASCII)
          _ 2. Translate print into braille
          _ 3. Format file prior to output
          _ 4. Output to embosser or printer
          _ 5. Global search and replace
          _ 6. Back translate braille into inkprint
          _ 7. Quit
```

Figure 4.

To take text from an ASCII textfile to braille the user would have to use options 1 through 4. A cautious user may actually want to make the computer perform one command at a time by pulling down the steps one at a time, but most users wishing to translate print into braille would type the following batch command: DOTS1234 filename.art, LPT1 and a stored encyclopedia article (filename.art) will be translated from ASCII to braille, formatted and printed out on a braille device (LPT1). Note it is necessary to format braille because braille characters take up more paper space than standard print, and the ASCII notations must be moved to accommodate for this factor.

The following is an actual example of a search and translation of an article found by a braille user in a CD-ROM encyclopedia and translated into braille format:

1. The patron found an article on asteroids and saved it on the hard disk, calling it aster.art and returned to DOS.
2. At the DOS prompt he called up the dots program by typing "Dots" at the dos prompt, e.g., C:\>dots
3. When the Dots program is loaded and dots menu appears (see Figure 5) s/he types: Dots1234 aster.art, LPT1 and in a matter of a few minutes the article is printed in braille.

If the patron is using a computer without a braille printer, but has access to one, s/he would follow steps 1 and 2 but when the Dots menu is loaded, s/he would substitute the following for Step 3:

3a. Type: Dots123 aster.art, A: to transfer the translated and formatted article to a diskette s/he had placed in the A drive.

Overall the program is easy to use and the results yield fairly good braille. It is considered by many braille users one of the top programs available. In previous releases the "global search and replace" option was not easy to use for the occasional user. It was necessary to use this option if you were trying to print something that has unrecognizable items like a word processor's "carriage return" notation still in the document. In the new release, however, 30 different word processors are recognized which will make the job easier. For instance in translating an article that is in column format, the user could import the document into his word processor and use the word processor's translator to take it to ASCII or use Hotdots search and replace option and answer the questions as:

1. Rule File? type "Global" then answer
2. Input? type "filename" and
3. Output? type "space.rule"

This rule will tell dots to erase all the spaces except the normal space of one. Raised Dots does offer technical assistance service to registered users (it offered the solution to the spacing problem, rather than the reference manual). The unique thing about this technical assistance line is that there is usually someone staffing it who will talk to you when you call! The assistants are always pleasant and try to be of help. The assistants are all "professional" Hotdots users themselves and know the shortcuts as well as solutions to program bugs that may surface. Raised Dots also publishes a self-titled, bimonthly newsletter (first year is free with software purchase) with helpful hints and readers' experiences. This newsletter also announces/reviews new computer apparatus as it becomes available in order to keep its readers up-to-date on new technology that can help them grow.

PC Braille

PC Braille is a product of ARTS Computer Products, Inc. Upon opening the user's guide one gets a short education on the subject of braille as well as enough information to sit down and use the translating program. In the beginning, the instruction book assumes you are a first-time user but expects you to have some DOS background by the time you are ready to actually print the braille (i.e., you are aware of what a DOS prompt is, you know what the "Print" command is, etc.).

The actual program, which produces a good translation,[6] could not be easier. After the program is loaded onto the hard disk, you simply type one direct command and in a matter of minutes you are translating a text file into braille (note: text files have no format and do not contain word processing codes). The command schema is as follows (using the article we saved on asteroids, aster.art):

1. At the DOS prompt type the following: C>bt -pbrailler aster.art >com1
2. Press the return key and formatted braille will begin to print.

When the program is done it will return you to the DOS prompt. This entire process takes only a few minutes. If you are translating a document with codes from a word processing program you may use the word processing program to translate it to ASCII and then translate it to braille. However, if you are taking something off an electronic bulletin board, or CD-ROM text which has multiple blank lines or multiple screen decorations such as ***'s, you will have to purchase another program to get rid of them. The program which works with PC Braille to take your file to a text file state is PC SIFT. The program literally looks through the entire file and removes the extra spaces and anything that doesn't follow the normal rules of spelling and formatting. This takes only one command: C> PC SIFT filename.art.

When you are returned to the DOS prompt, you simply move to the braille translator and type in the batch command to translate. Both the PC Sift and the PC Braille are automatic translators, that is, they will take general rules and translate them to a readable state, which will meet the NLS transcription standards. If you want to produce more accurate braille, the rules become more complicated.

To print your braille (PC Braille allows you to save the translations to disk, if a printer is not available) from its translated state, you will have to refer to your printer manual for answers to questions such as: device control, width and length of page, paper format and stock type. There is not a "hit list" or brailler to chose from as in some translator programs. The user's manual wisely suggests that a batch command be established to answer all these questions and to tell the brailler to print. A typical command line would be to type at the DOS prompt: C>bt -braillername %1>COM 1.

It is assumed that all the information on the brailler has been stored somewhere on your hard disk where it can be retrieved using this command. The user's manual suggests that users consult their DOS manual or contact the manufacturer or dealer if they do not know how to create a batch file.

Duxbury Braille Translator

The Duxbury braille translator is one of the most established translation programs in existence. It is a product of Duxbury Systems, which has local representatives, and it is also distributed by LS & S. In addition to translating English to braille in a highly efficient manner,[7] the Duxbury will also translate contracted Spanish and French, which is a help in an institution of higher learning where students and researchers may have to access foreign texts.

The basic instruction manual (there is also a five-volume manual available which contains the complete documentation for every rule used) is straightforward and cuts to the basic. It strongly suggests that the user have some rudimentary knowledge of the MS-DOS operating system, or at least the assistance of a person with such knowledge. Most of the terms Duxbury expects the user to know are already a part of our vocabulary (disk, file, prompt), so the instructions are clear.

The basic program is user-friendly and walks you through each step. After the translator is stored on the hard disk you can proceed to translate (Duxbury suggests that you do not work within the Duxbury directory, but create a work area so as not to corrupt the translator). At the DOS prompt you type: C> duxb, after which you will see a list (not a menu) of batch options, such as braille, format braille, ink, etc. These are listed simply for reference and one can get more information about any option at this starting point.

Duxbury assumes that most users will be taking print (ASCII) to formatted braille or braille to inkprint, and has paper size, pitch, and standard defaults programmed. Using the example of the same stored article on asteroids (aster.art) one would type:

1. *Braille aster.art*, assuming the paper length is equivalent to 25 lines and the width is 40 braille spaces. If this is not the case, you must type the correct numbers after the braille filename command. When the program is done translating you will be returned to the MS-DOS prompt. You are now ready to print or copy the translated text to disk. The formatted braille now has a .brf extension, so to print you will type the following command (the extension is the leader):
2. *Brfout aster*. You will then be asked the destination of the output (you can set up a default in your autoexec.bat file), which you will answer either with your printer's destination or disk drive's name. The copy will be made appropriately and then the program will proceed to set the number of copies you want, as well as answer questions on paper type. Many braille printers will allow you to set them up to default to your normal operating mode, which will allow you to skip these questions. The Duxbury also presumes that you are able to choose the following options on the printer to produce perfectly formatted braille: 1) select North American code; 2) turn off Grade I braille option; 3) turn off "word wrap" or "auto wraparound" option; 4) turn off "auto carriage return"; 5) turn off "auto line feed"; 6) set page length and width to their maximum values. If you are not able to choose these options, the program will still work, it simply will not be perfect.

	Does translation follow the Grade II translation rules according to Braille Assoc of North Am.?	Does it translate all documents?	Menu driven	Batch commands possible	Speed/ accuracy	Price
Hotdots	YES	YES	YES	YES	Y/Y	$350
PC Braille	YES	YES	NO	YES	Y/Y	$495+$180 for PC software +$180 for word processor software
Duxbury	YES	YES	YES	YES	Y/Y	$495

Figure 5. All software braille translators are relatively accurate and easy to use.

This discussion of the Duxbury translator was for the novice mode or the "fully prompted" and "parameter line" mode. For these modes, the user is answering questions or giving batch commands line by line. As the user becomes more familiar with the translator he or she can set up a batch file, write exceptions and generally save a lot of time and get 100 percent accurate braille translations (remember the five-volume set of exceptions). However, for most of us the above instructions are all that's needed to render a readable braille document.

Hardware Braille Translator

A hardware braille translator is a possible solution for the library which does not want to load another memory-resident program to an already over-taxed hard disk drive. There is only one brand currently available (imported from Australia), the Ransley Braille Interface (RBI), which is distributed by HumanWare and the L S & S Group. The device is priced at under $1,000 and weighs only eighteen ounces!

The Ransley connects to either a computer or a braille embosser and comes equipped with both serial and parallel ports (as well as a 9 volt DC adapter). The user wishing to translate standard printed text to braille simply types "!!E" at the end of the file he or she wants translated, pushes a button and in minutes the Grade II braille equivalent of the text is being printed, albeit to default settings. While this is the easy way to get braille translated, the user is also offered the options of setting page width and length as well as page numbering and margin settings or even to translate to Grade I braille as opposed to Grade II braille.

The Ransley does have a 24K buffer which makes it possible to temporarily store a small amount of text to be printed later. This unique peripheral is guaranteed for one year.

Braille n' Speak

Braille n' Speak (see page 32) can also be used as a "pseudo" braille translator. The unit can store information as braille text for future printing and eliminates the need for a software program, if the user is fluent in braille.

Braille Embossers

A braille embosser is definitely needed if braille hardcopy is desired. The embosser is, in simple terms, a printer that actually has braille cell "keys" which hit the printer paper hard enough to cause the paper to raise and make an impression where it was hit. There are quite a few braille embossers or printers on the market whose costs run from relatively inexpensive (under $1,000) to very expensive ($5,000). The difference in the costs can be attributed to speed of printing, the intensity of emboss strike, whether or not the machine will produce normal type as well as braille and the noise level of the actual printing process. If finding an inexpensive embosser is your goal, most braille users would not mind the softer or sharper dots (except those users with "less sensitive fingers," e.g., diabetics) or the longer wait to get their information printed in braille, but be aware that some of the sounds produced by a braille printer are louder than the loudest dot matrix printer—staff and people studying would definitely be disturbed by a noisy braille embosser.[8] It is suggested that a sound hood be installed on any embosser you may decide to purchase and that you buy the embosser from a company willing to service the machine for you and ship you a loaner machine while it is repairing the machine as it is impossible to find a local service person who is capable of fixing the equipment, even in metropolitan areas.

Standard-Sized

The following printers were evaluated by the American Foundation for the Blind's National Technology Center in 1987 and are still available. The criteria used in the evaluation were stringent and perhaps more detailed than most of us would demand of a standard printer. First measured was the speed of braille production per page of braille, then the noise level using a Simpson Model 886 sound-level meter. The quality of the embossed dots was measured against NLS standards.[9] They are all serviceable enough to withstand heavy use.

Index. The Index embosser produces high-quality braille, and patrons who are asked for their opinion of it are quite surprised when they are told it comes from a small braille printer. The patrons contacted in the aforementioned survey thought the quality of the braille (height of dots, consistency of the braille and the spacing between the lines) was excellent.[10]

The original Index was extremely noisy (72-77 decibels)[11] and made a noise on startup akin to an aircraft taking off. The newer model in current production is much quieter, produces braille twice as quickly (can print at up to 50 characters per second) and has added features such as horizontal printing and graphics spacing. The paper feed, however, is a factor to be dealt with. While you can purchase paper for this printer from several sources (not so with another brand), it is hard to get the paper under the bar and on its way to the tractor pins. Once through, the paper will flow easily if you allow the paper a drop of about 18".

The machine requires a few standard manipulations via rocker switches (i.e., top of form, online, print, edit) to adjust the impressions (see Figure 6). Once these are adjusted (the instruction manual has clear pictures of the switch positions), all the user has to do is give the computer the DOS command to print. This printer has a buffer large enough to hold the equivalent of 99 pages of information, which allows the user to move on to another topic while the information is being printed.

The Index embosser, while an excellent printer, has a rather confusing history. The machine is manufactured in Sweden and was originally imported by a company which is now part of TSI. TSI will maintain and sell reconditioned models of the older units which it calls MBOSS (these carry a limited warranty but are a good value at under $3,000). The newer models are sold by HumanWare and L S & S for between $3,000-$4,000, depending on the speed of braille printing.

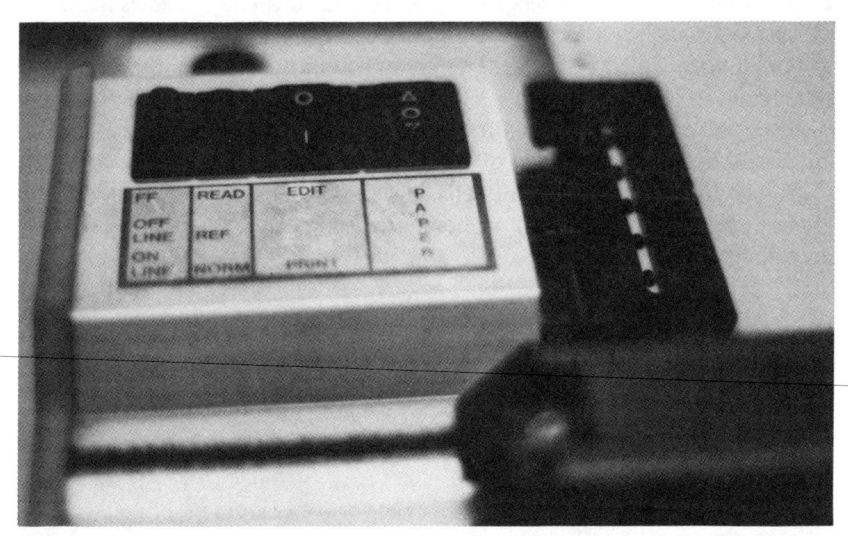

Figure 6. Toggle switches control the printer as the paper goes through the tractor feed.

Ohtsuki . The Ohtsuki printer is manufactured by Ohtsuki Communications Products, Inc. (which also makes commercial printers) and is distributed by both American Thermaform, Inc. and the LS & S Group. This printer stands alone in one way—it can print both braille and standard print at the same time (or print either format at will)! The plus of this feature is that a sighted person without any knowledge of braille can determine if the braille is translating correctly by reading the dot-matrix produced version (produced by an ink-roller rather than a ribbon), which for some users may make up for its deficits. The Ohtsuki is a rather quiet printer, measuring only 52dB to 58dB when in the braille mode. [12] Another plus is that the Ohtsuki has a built-in Grade II translation program that enables 6-dot braille to be translated into print. These features make it worth considering for the library environment where noise and space usage are concerns. The paper is relatively easy to load, but it uses notched, continuous-form paper available only through an Ohtsuki distributor.

The printer is not without faults, however. It requires some understanding of Basic programming language unless one is using the "demo" disk (a tutor). While the demo disk is easy to load there still exists many escape sequence commands which must be typed exactly before the printer will work. For example pressing: <esc> 1 T- will set the output lines spacing so that 25 lines of braille and print will fit on a page; pressing <esc> B will set the printer for braille only. Blind users found the machine difficult to use as the printer uses dip switches to change parameters and these dip switches are located behind a plate which needs to be pried off with a screwdriver.[13] The printer was found to be relatively slow and printed braille at 11 to 13 characters per second.[14] The braille produced met the standards set by the Library of Congress specifications for height of dots, base of diameter, and center-to-center corresponding dots of adjacent cells, but the cell spacing was significantly higher (.003-.012 of an inch) when adjacent dots within the same cell were measured center to center.

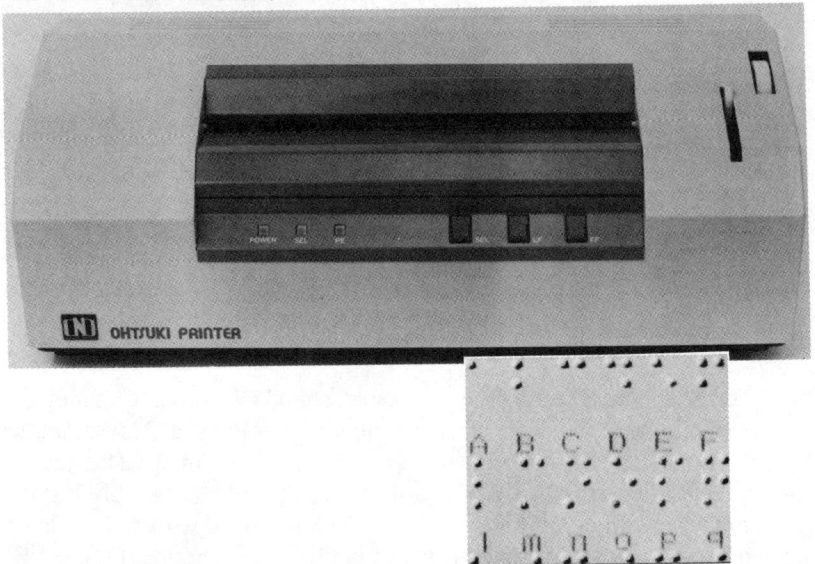

Figure 7. The Ohtsuki printer is the only printer that will print conventional print and braille.

Actual respondents in the survey did not feel that the spacing between the lines was adequate and overall felt that this printer created poor grade of braille even though it passed most of the tests.[15]

The printer comes with both a parallel and a serial interface card. Users suggest that a parallel interface be used with switches set to: on on off on off off.[16] This allows printing with less manipulation. If working from a braille translating program, you can avoid the problem of typing a long escape sequence by simply choosing the Ohtsuki from the menu of printers, choosing the "online" command from the printer mode choices (SEL button).[17] While the latter solution to the problem sounds simple enough, be aware that the Ohtsuki does not have a buffer, and that the entire process may hang up translation too long.

The warranty on the machine is six months with an option for an extended limited warranty. The warranty covers a loaner option which is reasonable for a printer as compact as this one (size 20.5 x 6 .8 x 10.6 inches) which weighs only 24 lbs. The consumers testing this model did appreciate its compactness.[18]

VersaPoint-40. Manufactured by TeleSensory Products Inc. (TSI) and distributed by TSI and Raised Dots Computing, VersaPoint-40 offers the consumer a medium-priced braille embosser ($3,500) which produces braille quickly (40 characters per second) and effectively (consumers found the braille had problems but was acceptable).[19] The VersaPoint is an adaptable embosser as it will connect with either a serial port or a parallel port, allowing the user to start printing anywhere on the page and print either vertically or horizontally (the horizontal option is a plus if the user wants the information printed exactly as it is displayed on the screen, rather that being reformatted as it must be when using the portrait format).

The noise level was the thing that had to be reckoned with as the noise range fell between 70dB-75dBs (decibel level not available on current model). The consumers testing model BP 1A had said it sounded like a machine gun in both volume and quality of sound and had a hammering sound that could be distracting to others in the area.[20] The manufacturer had promised that other models would be quieter and upon listening to the current model, it is agreed that TeleSensory held to its pledge as the hammering noise is all but gone. The braille is now created with solenoids, each only having to braille four cells per line to reduce strain on the embossing heads.[21] Each generation of this company's machines is improved and it does strive to correct problems.

The paperfeed is relatively easy to use—simply push the line-feed button and read button in at the same time and the tractor feed device will advance the paper smoothly; additionally it will reverse the paper so that the user can review what is being printed.

The VersaPoint has an extremely large buffer (30k) which allows you to dump the document you wish to print into the embosser and continue to work on the next project. Another plus of this printer is that it can store up to five parameter settings. The printer comes programmed with the five most common configurations which aid the novice braille embosser user as one of them is a configuration to take print to braille. Simply choose the configuration you wish to use from a control panel and you are printing in that format in a matter of seconds without even going through a software translator.

VersaPoint-40 is a welcomed upgrade to the VersaPoint Model BP 1A, which was the model evaluated in the study conducted by the AFB. It now carries a one-year warranty (with extended warranties offered) and is part of the TSI network, whose representatives are always willing to do a demonstration for you as well as offering a toll-free number for technical assistance. VersaPoint was the printer of choice in the American Foundation for the Blind's study.[22]

Romeo. Produced and distributed by Enabling Technologies, the Romeo can be called the bargain of the lot, as its cost is approximately $3,000. It is comparatively small (20 x 13 x 6) and even has its own carrying case. The Romeo printer will accept either a serial or a parallel, and prints at a rate of 20 characters per second. The paper feed is relatively easy to use, although the tractor-fed paper is sometimes difficult to guide through the platen.[23] Using the printer is not difficult as all commands are given through a keypad, similar to that of a hand-held calculator. Parameters for printing can be set to one of 16 menus. The Romeo does not have an internal braille translator.

The noise level was found to be between 59dB to 65dB but the noise produced was not an irritating one.[24] One "noise" to note however is the signal that the printer gives when it runs its self-test and all is found to be OK — the first few notes from Romeo and Juliet (if the test fails, the first few notes of Chopin's funeral dirge are heard). While cute the first few times through, this can become tiresome.

The quality of braille produced by Romeo is acceptable according to the standards of the Library of Congress. The evaluators found the criterion used to measure line spacing was off by .006 inch, but that the spacing between cells was good and the dots sharp and consistent.

There is also an upgraded version of Romeo available, which prints twice as fast. Both carry a 90-day warranty with an extended yearly service contract available. This is a good choice if you are looking for a printer that can be tucked to the side when not being used as it is relatively small (the carrying case also makes loaning to students possible).

Deluxe

Pixelmaster 2. Pixelmaster 2, manufactured by Howtek and available from American Thermoform, L S & S and Howtek, is not in the same class as the previously mentioned braille embossers. Pixelmaster 2 is an expensive printer ($7,000), but if price is no object Pixelmaster presents the user with features that will astound and presents such an impressive document that "fund-raising" letters could be printed using it. In addition to quietly printing braille using raised ink, this printer will print maps, charts, images, conventional print (in any one of 35 common laser fonts) and translate text stored as ASCII files into braille.

Howtek uses a "thermal jetting" technology to produce raised dots or lines on standard paper. The enhanced dots (or lines) are made of ink which is plastic based, heated high enough to melt and precisely flows through the jets and onto the paper. The ink solidifies instantaneously when it comes into contact with the paper. The dot or line formed is not as crisp as one that has actually been struck out by an embosser, but can be read by those who have good sensitivity in their fingertips.

Howtek worked closely with the National Federation of the Blind to produce the graphic/text printer in order that it would adhere to standards. The Federation evidently was pleased with the product as it used the Pixelmaster to produce floor plans for the attendees of its National Convention in the summer of 1990.[25]

This printer is one that would serve as a bridge of understanding between the non-impaired user and the visually impaired and blind computer user. It would also help the impaired user, who had some vision and knew how and where to look, understand (by touch) diagrams and illustrations that sometimes cannot fully be described. Where it falls short is in helping the blind user who has not had map reading or has never had any training in depth perception because it actually has too much detail. Figure 8 is a copy of an illustration that was printed using the ink jets; each line was raised. A totally blind patron who had never seen a sailboat was able to run his fingers over it and determine the ship's sails in relation to its bow.

Conclusion

Offering braille access to information is an exciting challenge and one which will not go unrewarded for the efforts and dollars expended. Barbara Wegreich is a senior programmer at Wang Laboratories who uses a paperless braille display to conduct "life." She says that the PC with its adaptive braille technology is her lifeline and through it she is able to access computer services such as CompuServe or Delphi as well as learn new things

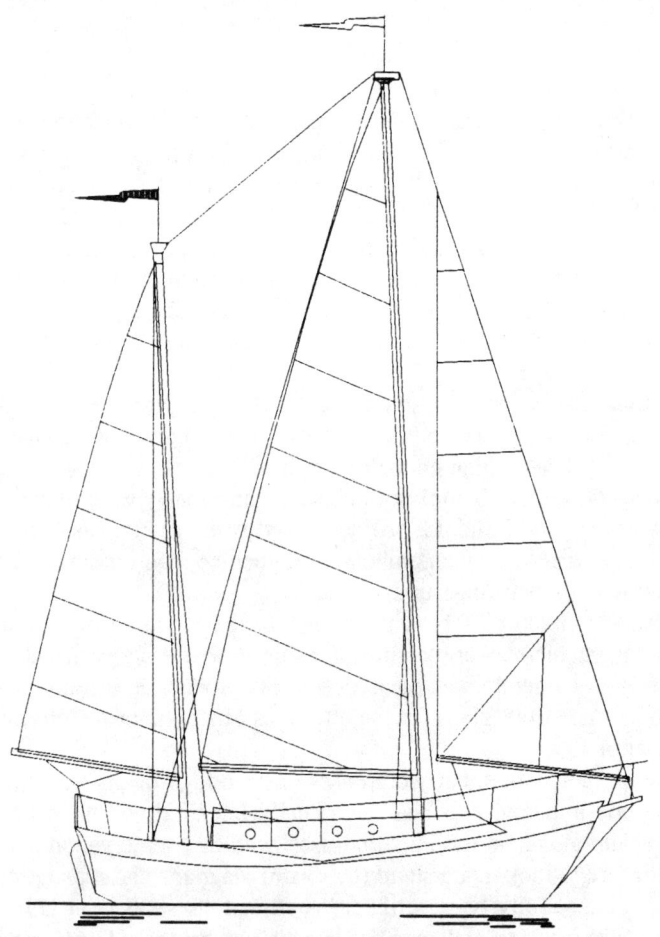

46 *Library Technology for Visually and Physically Impaired Patrons*

Figure 8. *The original copy of this features slightly raised sails and allows the blind or visually impaired user to feel the image.*

using any "off-the-shelf" computer product whenever she wants to (as opposed to when someone translates it for her).[26]

Even if the equipment or software you purchase serves only one blind patron, you are giving that person what he or she is entitled to—the same access to information that a sighted person has.

4

Audio Output

Background Information

The ability to get audio output via computers has been in existence for over a decade. One of the original and more famous pioneers in the field was Raymond Kurzweil who in 1976 produced an elaborate computer scanning system which after many manipulations (and a lot of luck) read aloud certain printed texts using synthetic speech. This pioneering unit was expensive, difficult to use and temperamental, but paved the way for a variety of devices that will read aloud personal computer screens/video display terminals or printed texts.[1]

The first generation of speech synthesizers was not easy to understand and did not allow the user to adjust items indicative to speech patterns (pitch, speed, etc.). This is changing rapidly and each generation of synthesizers brings forth voices which are easier to understand and more "human" sounding. As a result we are hearing more synthetic speech in our living space such as service vending machines selling lottery tickets; diagnostic machines in hospitals which use synthesizers to keep staff from possible overexposure to radiation; even the Atlanta International Airport uses Kurzweil synthetics to give directions to passengers. The fact remains, however, that synthesized speech is still just that and, for a percentage of the population, not an acceptable substitute for a voice.

The population which expresses difficulty with synthetic speech in general is the same group that has a difficult time hearing or understanding the spoken word by a human being who is properly enunciating words and speaking loudly. The speech access program reads text following general grammatical rules. As the English language is rather complex and filled with exceptions, syllable emphasis is not always possible and mispronunciations common. The savvy personal computer user, however, knows the screen readers' limits and knows when to repeat text or spell a word aloud letter-by-letter so that he or she will know what the word is (rather than skipping it). This skilled user also knows the commands to give to the screen reader to ignore graphics and read items within windows and is perfectly satisfied with the speech of the computer.

An adept computer user will know how to scan text properly (like any scanner, it is necessary to scan text at a certain speed and smoothness to get a good readout) or be able to learn, while a person who fears technology will be afraid to try to scan text.

The occasional user who does not take the time to learn how to use either a screen reading program or a text scanner will quickly become disillusioned with synthetic speech, which is unfortunate, as it is for some (non-braille or large-print readers) the only alternative to accessing information.

Audio output also benefits those who have learning disabilities which require a multi-sensory approach to learning. Being able to hear text as well as see the text helps this portion of the population learn as both the auditory and visual portions of the brain are stimulated simultaneously. This approach also allows the person to hear and see the text as many times as necessary to learn without asking a tutor (who has limited time and patience) to do the same.

What It Involves

Synthetic speech is comprised of two main elements: the synthesizer that physically produces the speech and the software program that interacts with the computer and the application program.[2] If you are not purchasing a self-contained unit be aware that the software program must be compatible with the synthesizer that it is to drive. Figure 1 is an example of how the basic system operates.

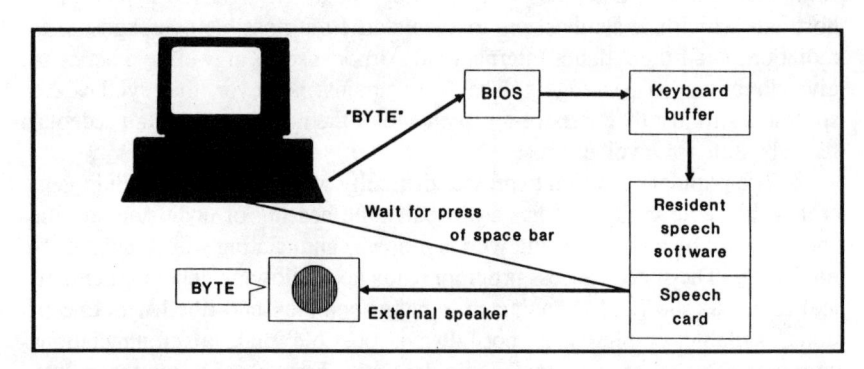

Figure 1. A speech synthesis system usually consists of resident software (screen reader), a speech-synthesis board with audio amplification, and a speaker. When the user types on the keyboard, the system turns the letters into phonemes, runs through a series of rules that tell it how to say the word, and outputs the word through the speaker. Source: Joe Lazzaro, "Opening Doors for the Disabled," BYTE, August 1990.

Acceptable audio output is possible without expending a large amount of money or instructional time. Audio output can be as simple as the software driver and synthesizer installation you provide for a standard computer; medium ranged such as the special purchase of a peripheral designed for screen reading; or as elaborate as a text scanner, which would make much printed text accessible.

Choosing the appropriate speech access method depends on the applications you wish to use it with and the patron group you perceive as using it. If you are going to use it on a personal computer you need only look for a software driver that will work with personal computers, but if you are going to go online you must choose a driver that will work in a mainframe environment.

Be aware of the following: whatever route you decide to go there are operating variances within each and numerous programs available; most of the screen readers will also have more features than you will need, as they were developed for use with application programs such as word processors; and users of the synthesizers have their favorites as do users of word processing programs, so it is impossible to choose one that all users will like.

There are certain basic features to look for in any speech program:[3]

1. Reading the current, previous, and nest characters as well as words, lines, sentences and paragraphs selectively.
2. The identifications of various positions on the screen (i.e., grid location—line, row, and column).
3. The ease by which movement can be made around the screen.
4. The number and configuration of keystrokes required to implement the function.
5. The ability to control speech (i.e., volume, pitch, rate).
6. The ability to monitor screen changes (error messages, status).
7. Use of macros.
8. Difficulty of installation, clarity of documentation and availability/quality of online help facilities.

Software Drivers for Synthesizers

The speech-to-text synthesizer drivers that are discussed in this section were either evaluated by the National Technology Center of the American Foundation for the Blind or actual users contacted by the National Braille Press.[4] These drivers tell the synthesizer what to do and how to do it; they are to the speech synthesizer what the brain is to the mouth. The software drivers are all priced at around $500 and are needed for screen access—without them, the synthesizer would read the screen text word by word. As mentioned, you will find that most synthesizer users will swear that the one they use is the best, so it is suggested that you find the one that you consider the easiest to learn at the price you can afford. If money is a factor, be aware that there are a few "shareware" synthesizer-drivers in the public domain. If you need to save the cost of a driver to purchase the synthesizer, one of these will do (ease of operation, quality of reading will not be the same) and can be acquired through user networks for the disabled or free from some dealers with the purchase of another product.

Artic Visions

Artic Visions, produced by Artic Technologies, can turn any personal computer into one that is able to read aloud virtually any text that appears on the screen or is stored on disk. It costs approximately $500 and is available directly from Artic Technologies, as well as a number of strategically located representatives. It offers a technical assistance helpline and publishes a newsletter with technical hints.

Artic Visions will drive only one speech board, a SynPhonix Vision Enhanced Speech Translator (VEST), a speech synthesizer board with microphone which must be slipped into an open slot in the chassis. The Artic "driving" software is then installed on the hard drive as a memory-resident program. Artic Visions' software limitations in regard to compatible synthesizers can be seen as both an advantage and a disadvantage. The advantage is that since the driver was designed for the board it has complete control over it and does not have to make allowances for "nuances" of other brands of synthesizers.[5] The disadvantage is that you are locked into purchasing VEST and, should you not like the speech output, you would have to purchase both a new synthesizer and a new driver. This package allows you the option of installing a turbo foot pedal that will aid the user in reading and re-reading on screen text at different speeds without having to enter commands with the keypad. This is helpful to those with limited usage of their hands as well as those who really want speed in their reader.

Once the driver and board are installed, all that needs to be done to get voice output is for the user to type at the DOS prompt the following command: C:\av and the program begins to read everything that appears on the screen including the DOS information. The program will use the default settings as far as pitch, speed and volume are concerned because it comes up in the AP-TRACK (application tracking) mode. These qualities can easily be changed by entering the "REVIEW" mode which makes use of five different voice channels! This allows the user, for instance, to listen to the unknown text on the screen at a slower rate of speed and the known keyboard input at a faster rate and screen locators at still another.

```
C>AVISION

           VISIONS ENHANCED SPEECH TRANSLATOR

    SPECIAL RELEASE FOR ARTIC VISIONS
    (C)COPYRIGHT 1984, 1985, 1988, 1989
    BY ARTIC TECHNOLOGIES
    ALL RIGHTS RESERVED

       S/N 56032XX          VEST VER 1.20 ENGLISH

C>AVISION
               ARTIC VISION    2

    VOICE OUTPUT COMPUTER ACCESS SYTEM
    (c)COPYRIGHT 1986, 1987, 1990
    BY ARTIC TECHNOLOGIES.
    ALL RIGHTS RESERVED.

       S/N 56032XX      VERSION 2.20
```

Figure 2. After loading the software, the screen will immediately start to be read. The user will make any needed adjustments for pitch, speed, and loudness.

Pressing "scroll lock" will take you to the Review mode, in which the user is able to tell the synthesizer how to enunciate a word correctly or change the pitch. The pitch is changed by pressing "ALT R" to get into the menu and then pressing P and a number from 0-9 (the pitch numbers can be sampled by pressing the space bar and up arrow or down arrow). If a user has any question of how a word is spelled or the context in which it is being used, the review mode will take him or her through the word letter by letter or word by word, until a clear understanding is made. These prompts are also controlled by key combinations such as "ALT PG DN" to read the current word (note this feature, as well as 11 others, can be accessed in AP-TRACK).

For the user who quickly wishes to scan an article of text, and is not familiar enough with the procedures of Artic (i.e., to make a window(s) and direct the reader to read only text in that grid), this memory-resident program can be called up and used with the DOS command of "TYPE" to read stored text in an uninterrupted flow, which is perfect for reading items such as encyclopedia articles.

The turbo-pedal mentioned above as an option will move the user through text quickly as will a recently added hardware device called the Gizmo. Gizmo allows the user to move through the text without using the main keyboard, making it easier to learn the basic combination of keys that make this driver so powerful. Gizmo is a welcome addition to the Artic family as it allows the user to program macros for individual applications that will take him through text more directly (i.e., the program is not reliant on the computer's keyboard). Gizmo's features are also of help to the occasional user if access points to titles can be pre-programmed by someone versed in Artic usage. This may aid the physically disabled who experience trouble with executing some of the commands. Having a separate control pad also eliminates problems of certain function keys interfering with the programs (e.g., some ALT functions of Visions cause conflicts with off-the-shelf application programs which use ALT functions heavily) which was the only criticism users had of Artic Visions.[6] (Note: this is the same Gizmo used with Artic's Focus large-print program; one unit can control both programs.)

Flipper

Flipper is a software synthesizer driver produced and distributed by Omnichron Corp. and priced significantly under $500. Flipper gives the user the option of working with several different brands of speech cards (Artic SynPhonix, AICOM Accent SA Turbo and Votrax Votalker) as well as external synthesizers such as AICOM Accent SA Turbo, Audapter, DECtalk, Echo and Votrax personal speech system. Flipper will also work in the mainframe, (IRMA-type) environment.

Flipper's basic functions are relatively easy to use and uniquely require no previous computer skills.[7] This ease starts with the installation procedure which consists of installing either an internal card synthesizer or an external device (special instructions are given for these), then loading Flipper to your hard drive (or floppy disk drive), a procedure which takes only minutes and begins with the user typing "INSTALL." The voice output is immediate and begins with synthesized instructions for continuing the installation.

Flipper does have two modes of user operation: a "regular" mode which is the application mode (also the default mode) and a "review" mode which is the mode in which most users versed in the intricacies of Flipper use to read the screen. Review mode is accessed by simply by pressing the: ALT key and typing a ";" (semicolon).

The regular mode has enough keyboard commands (logical in their assignment) to let a user breeze through a screen reading; this is done with the "Quick Keyboard Command" functions. Many of these functions rely on the use of the "ALT" key and various keys around the "home row" keys. Some examples of the simplicity of the commands to give to the synthesizer are as follows:

- to read the sentence above the cursor press ALT and "U"
- to read the current sentence press ALT and "I"
- to read the sentence below the cursor press ALT and "O"
- to read the word to the left of the cursor press ALT and "J"
- to read the word to the right of the cursor press ALT and "K"
- to read the word under the cursor press ALT and "L"
- to read the entire page press ALT and "P"

The review mode encompasses all these commands and adds quite a few features such as screen reading customizing and the ability to have the time announced (ALT "T"). The customizing allows the user to make choices among 42 predetermined options as to how the screen reader will save, load, react to punctuation, begin to read, etc. What makes Flipper different is that the user is able to save the primary configuration as well as secondary configurations he or she likes using the "Flipsave" application for future use (either on a personal diskette or named and stored on the hard disk, if space allows using a named file). The program also allows the user to "flip" back and forth between applications if desired. If the user wishes to print information from the screen using an attached electronic brailler, there is a "flip" feature that allows him to do this (a line at a time if desired) as the screen is being read.

The overall consensus is that Flipper is a good software driver for the occasional user because it is logical and easy to learn.[8] It has an easily accessible "help" feature in the review mode which will tell the user the function of the key press, thus saving staff from numerous queries.

Jaws (Jobs Access with Speech)

JAWS is produced by Henter-Joyce, whose company logo boldly announces the company as the "Experts in Access Technology." This software synthesizer driver was developed by Henter-Joyce with input from users and training centers such as the Trace Center. The program, costing approximately $500, is sold both through the manufacturer and the L S & S Group and comes with a one-year limited warranty.

JAWS will work with most text-to-speech synthesizers, in particular, Accent, Artic SynPhonix, Echo, Votalker, and DECtalk. Of the speech access programs evaluated in the 1990 study by the National Technology Center, American Foundation for the Blind,[9] JAWS was deemed the easiest to learn and operate. The study went so far as to say that learning it was actually "fun." The installation is as easy as typing "INSTALL" and answering a few questions concerning the speech synthesizer being used (the JAWS manual actually has instructions on how to install the boards, which other companies manufacture).

JAWS is the only text-to-speech translator that has a pop-up menu system which makes it easy to use the program. The menu system is logical and consistent using a four-line deep offering throughout. The screen reading functions were all built around the menus, which helps the user to learn them easily. Figure 3 illustrates the sensibility of the menu system as the user does not have to memorize needed procedures.

Another reason why JAWS is an easy program to learn is that Henter-Joyce kept in mind that all computer keyboards are not standard and that while the "alpha" and "function" keys were not necessarily in the same location on all keyboards, the numeric keypad, number row, as well as a few other keys were. They built all of JAWS function commands around this observation and as a result, almost all commonly used functions can be carried out using one hand (a plus for the physically impaired person as well) and the less common use of the menu which is easily accessed using a Hot Key.

Unlike other programs which require you to shift from one mode to another in order to change speech parameters, define 200 window parameters, and adjust universal parameters, such as the way words are pronounced, pause between words, etc., the user is able to do this through a menu. These menus, which are quickly called up, are a great help for the inexperienced user who does not have the time or does not want to take the time to learn yet another program. For the experts, who do not want a menu popping up whenever they wish to change functions, there is an option which disables the menus.

JAWS is a sophisticated screen reader that has features such as an Auto-Speak Macro, which will automatically perform tasks when it sees changes. These macros were written with the "if...then" logic which saves the user a lot of time and yields a better reading. Additionally JAWS is able to take advantage of a 16 color screen by recognizing and reporting the colors, which helps to create windows and report changes on the screen. The JAWS software driver also has its own cursor which is seen as an advantage if the user is accessing a program that actively uses a cursor.

JAWS will more than adequately suit the needs of the library user wishing to access reference works via a personal computer and speech synthe-

```
─────────────────────JAWS from menu─────────────────────
 Speak      Activate    Quiet     Revise    Monitor
 Speak a frame or rectangular section of screen
```

C>

Figure 3. JAWS menu system

sizer. JAWS has so many utilities and function possibilities that it is able to make the synthesizer do what the user wants it to when reading a screen. Its strongest points are its ease of use and the fact that it requires very little learning on the part of the librarian, the technical assistant or the patron. Henter-Joyce has a toll-free technical assistance line.

IBM Screen Reader

IBM Screen Reader is the only program developed by a major "mainstream" corporation (i.e., one that doesn't have as its corporate goal the rehabilitation of the disabled) specifically for the physically challenged. The IBM Screen Reader sells for slightly over $600 and has a one-year limited warranty. The package should be available by special order through your local IBM representative (or through IBM Special Needs Center) or the LS & S Group. It will work on any IBM PC model and should work on most true clones. It is sugggested that a demo be done on your particular model since developers at IBM were using specific IBM criteria and not allowing for varience.[10] The IBM Screen Reader does have versatility in regard to speech synthesizers and will work with the following: Accent, Apollo, Audapter, DECtalk, Echo PC, PSS and VoxBox.

What makes this software package special is that it actually comes with a piece of hardware which must be used to access the software. This hardware is a keypad which plugs into the mouse port of the computer. This keypad eliminates all key command conflicts between the reader and the application progam being read. Through this keypad the user can read and monitor the screen. The keypad has 12 numeric keys in the same layout as the buttons on a telephone and a column of letters "A through D" just to the right side of the keypad. The keypad also has two very important buttons: the "HELP" button and a "STOP" button. Basic commands are simple, for instance:

- pressing key "1" reads the line previous to the current line;
- keys "0B" give the color attributes of the character at the cursor;
- keys "025" will read line 25.

The more advanced workings of Screen Reader are not as easy to use, but allow an advanced user more power, as s/he is actually able to program undefined key sequences to his or her needs. The computer language used, although similar to "C" language or PASCAL, is unique to the Screen Reader and is called "Profile Access Language (PAL)."[11]

Once the user learns the fundamentals of PAL, s/he will be able to make the synthesizer:[12]

1. Speak special information from the screen.
2. Create reading windows; define and activate autospeaks (e.g., when a user is accessing a CD-ROM encyclopedia whose pages always hit the screen in the same place and whose option commands do as well, he or she can program IBM Screen Reader to begin reading at the given place(s) each time).
3. Dictate when to spell information (e.g., user could program the reader to spell words over three syllables or over 10 letters).
4. Change how the synthesizer speaks (e.g., pitch, rate).

If the user does not have any programming background learning PAL will be challenging.[13] Once learned, however, it becomes one of the most powerful screen readers available because it can respond to a long string of commands, which are called "profiles." Of help in creating "profiles" is a quarterly newsletter that contains tips and techniques. Also, the technical assistance help line is manned by visually impaired users, who can help create profiles to solve problems.

Screen Reader is an excellent program and worth considering if you intend it to be used in word processing-type programs as well as in reference-type situations. However, remember that what sets Screen Reader apart from other software synthesizer-drivers are its independent input keypad (only needed if reading screens which are part of other application programs, e.g., Lotus 1-2-3) and its user programming options (application profiles). These are the "extras" you are getting for your "extra" money. Additionally, the program will not work without the keypad—you must be willing to sacrifice a mouse port; and while the program will work straight out of the box, it's the application profiles that give it strength, and these require some programming background.[14]

Summary

Although this listing of software synthesizer drivers is by no means exhaustive, we have discussed a sampling of those which have had consumer feedback or have unique characteristics. Most software drivers on the marketplace (available through the sources listed in Appendix 2) will serve most needs adequately. Choose the one that will best suit the needs of your user group. If the user group is an academic one it will appreciate the IBM Screen Reader because it will allow it to use powerful commands; if the user group is a public one, it will appreciate an easy-to-learn program such as JAWS or

Flipper; if the user group is one that demands accuracy and pre-determined commands, then a program similar to Artic Visions would be the choice.

Text-to-Speech Synthesizers

The synthesizer is as important a part of the screen reader program as the driver, but easier to understand. You simply purchase and install a synthesizer card in an empty slot in your computer or attach a peripheral to an empty port. You will actually get voice output immediately from either. The option you select will be determined by the options open to you on your computer (i.e., is there an empty slot or port?). If choosing the card approach, be sure to check if it is available in the size that will fit the slot of your computer's chassis. The following synthesizers were evaluated by IBM[15] or consumers and are listed here because they are the most versatile and are compatible with the more popular software drivers. Be aware that there are many more good synthesizers available at competitive prices. There is a difference in voice quality among synthesizers, but in reality this difference is as subjective as the software driver. If you have access to a Macintosh, with Hypercard 1.0 or 2.0, it is well worth spending $25 to purchase a voice sampler from Trace Center (the Mac version is the only one currently available with an IBM version due in summer 1991). This sampler contains digitally recorded voice samples from major speech synthesizers so that they can be compared and evaluated more easily.

	Menu	Quick access	Mainframe Compatible	Two modes of operation	Macro driver	Compatible with multitude of speech cards	Separate cursor control	Cost
Artic	NO	NO	NO	YES	YES	NO	N (Y with Gizmo)	$500
Flipper	NO	YES	YES	YES	YES	YES	NO	$500
JAWS	YES	YES	NO	YES	YES	YES	YES	$500
IBM Screen Reader	NO	YES	NO	YES	YES	YES	YES	$600

Figure 4. Screen readers for speech synthesizers

Internal Synthesizers

Accent-PC. The Accent-PC synthesizer is distributed by AICOM corporation and the L S & S Group, and is priced at slightly under $1,000. Accent is a text-to-speech synthesizer with unlimited vocabulary capability (20,000 word dictionary). The synthesizer employs the standard text-to-speech processor which speaks in two modes—text and spell. Speech rate is extremely variable with the low end of the rate being 60 words per minute and the high end being 800 words per minute. This synthesizer also has an 8K byte text buffer which allows the reader to "digest" the information and output it in a readable manner. Technical support for Accent is available.

DECtalk. DECtalk is a full-featured voice synthesizer which offers the user a choice of nine voices (including a child's and four women's voices). The system is capable of reading aloud at the rate of 120 to 350 words per minute. DECtalk takes into consideration surrounding words and their effects on individual pronunciations. The unit also provides a user-specified dictionary of commonly used acronyms, trade names and special words. DECtalk may speak through its internal speaker, external speaker, headphones or "over-the-phone," which increases its usage.

The synthesizer is available through the Digital Equipment Corporation (DEC) and is popular enough (because it is used in commercial establishments) that a local representative would be able to give you information about the synthesizer. What he may not remember to tell you is that DEC has a DECtalk Grant Program available to non-profit organizations that service the handicapped (limited number available). DEC offers a 67 percent grant applicable toward the purchase of a DECtalk unit (which includes the personal computer with synthesizer) retailing at approximately $4,500. The applicant has to fill out a standard grant application but, if you are buying a personal computer specifically for the impaired, this is a good chance to get a quality synthesizer *and* a personal computer at under $2,000! DECtalk is incorporated in many other "talking" appliances and is the most popular voice used in such mainstream applications as banking functions.

Echo PC. There are various models of the Echo PC which are produced and distributed by Street Electronics and Western Center for Microcomputers in Special Education (also L S & S), all of which are economically priced at under $300. The Echo cards have been somewhat specialized in that Street Electronics has developed special cards for the more popular IBM clones which makes for a better link. The Echo synthesizers come with a text-to-speech software driver called Textalker, which has a small dictionary of 700 pre-recorded human-voiced words stored on a floppy disk, for use with application programs (a larger dictionary is available for the Echo for an additional $50). Echo's external speaker comes with a volume control. All models come with an item rather unique to synthesizers—a "game port," capable of interfacing with joy sticks or other types of alternate input devices. Although not a synthesizer that receives accolades from users (it has a highly robotic voice), it is serviceable (it will verbalize all off-the-shelf products including game packages) for the smaller budget.[16]

Prose 4000. Prose 4000 is a product of the Centigram Commnuication Corp. and is distributed by Centigram and L S & S Group. Priced at just under $2,000, Prose 4000 rides the high end of the synthesizer scale. Its attributes, however, make its purchase justified. It has a pronunciation accuracy of 99.4 percent on an industry standard test. Its speech rate varies from 50 to 250 words/minute and has an unlimited, variable pitch selection and attenuation. The user is also able to select one of three male voices to do the reading. Prose 4000 will work with IBM Screen Reader as well as other widely available packages.

SynPhonix. SynPhonix is produced and distributed by Artic Technologies and supported by area sales representatives. Price-wise, Artic at $500 is at the low end of the internal synthesizers. Artic Technologies has been producing and improving the SynPhonix synthesizer for the IBM PC since 1984. The cards have constantly been updated as technology advanced, thus they have a synthesizer card for just about any computer, including some laptops. All the cards have a speech chip (Artic-263 phoneme synthesizer) which is considered to be a hardware model of a human voice. Artic Technologies admits that there are other products that may sound more natural but maintains that its product is more accurate, which brings up a topic of debate (i.e., some who use the screen review for extended periods say accuracy is more important because it eliminates the need to re-read, while others say that they would rather listen to pleasant sounds twice as long than listen to irritating sounds once).

Syntha-Voice, Model I. Syntha-Voice, Model I is produced and distributed by Syntha-Voice Computers and is priced at approximately $600. This card is part of a family of synthesizers developed by a team of visually impaired and sighted programmers, engineers, and rehabilitation consultants. Although the Syntha-Voice was designed to work the company's software driver, Slimware,[17] it is user friendly to a number of software drivers. It has 8K of memory for storing a "users' vocabulary," which avoids any dependency on the computer for speech translation or memory. It will speak from 50 to 700 words per minute at one of eight pitch settings. The unique thing about Syntha-Voice is its ability to properly pronounce words with multiple possible pronunciations, such as "read," by taking these words in context. For example, most synthesizers would read the following sentence: "I read this yesterday and I will probably have to read it again tomorrow," as: "I {reed} this yesterday and I will probably {reed} this again tomorrow," rather than Syntha-Voice's "I {red} this yesterday and I will probably {reed} this again tomorrow."

Another feature that really should be applauded is an easy method to turn off screen display "glitz," for example, multiple **** or ——— as well as illustrations which really cause interruptions in most screen reading programs.

Nomad. Syntha-Voice is also incorporated into a self-contained portable computer unit that weighs nine pounds (complete with soft-driver) and is called "Nomad." Nomad is moderately priced at under $2,500, complete with modem. The Nomad is available with a standard or braille keyboard. The use of a braille keyboard allows the user to input information in braille and have it translated into standard print using a back translator.

External Speakers

Accent-SA. The Accent-SA synthesizer is distributed by AICOM Corporation and the L S & S Group, and is priced at slightly under $1,000. Like the Accent-PC, it is a text-to-speech synthesizer with unlimited vocabulary capability (20,000-word dictionary). In addition to emulating all of the other qualities of Accent-PC, it has the same lightning-quick response time (less than 20 milli-seconds in the "fast-processing" mode) to read commands. It also has the 8K buffer which will store approximately 500 10-character words. If surface space is a concern, it should be noted that this unit is sleek and measures only 5.5" x 11.5" x 1.6".

Apollo. The Apollo synthesizer is produced by Dolphin Systems of Worcester, England, and is distributed in the United States by Boston Information and Technology Corp. Although Apollo was originally designed to work with the software system called "HAL," it works well with the IBM Screen Reader and other popular drivers.[18] Apollo offers clear speech with pleasant inflection and tonal quality as well as variable pitch, intonation and voices. Its features include a quick response to speak and mute and 16 speeds from slow to very fast. This synthesizer is unique because it utilizes a digital signal processor, incorporating a mathematical model of sound qualities of throat and tongue to produce speech; the result is a more "human-like" quality of sound.

Audapter. Audapter, which sells for approximately $1,100, is produced and distributed by Personal Data Systems (also distributed by L S & S). This synthesizer's main attribute is indeed a noble one: it reads intelligibly over 93 percent of the time on the industry standard test (this is one of only a few synthesizers that reports its score). Another feature that makes it a special synthesizer is that it offers the user a simple menu, independent of a software driver, to alter the speech rate, voice, pitch and other parameters, and save them to non-volatile memory. It is compatible with many of the software drivers.

Personal Speech System (PSS). The Personal Speech System (PSS), priced at $500, is one of several quality synthesizers produced and distributed by Votrax Inc. (also distributed by L S & S). This unit is self-contained and allows the user to correct mispronounced words either by standard orthographic or special phonetic spellings. It has a large buffer of 3,500 characters and the standard features of speech rate, intonation, amplitude adjustment. What makes PSS unique, however, is the fact that it is able to produce sound effects/music with voice mixing simultaneously, which is a plus if usage plans involve interfacing with CD-ROM units which may be using multimedia materials. PSS is extremely adaptable as connector cables are available for virtually every IBM PC clone on the market and can be connected to a

	Screen Clear	2 Modes: Read/spell	Words/ minute	Buffer	Compatible	Cost
Accent PC	NO	YES	60-800	YES	YES	$1000
DECTalk	NO	YES	120-350	YES	YES	$4500
Echo PC	NO	YES	ADJUSTABLE	YES	YES	$250
Prose 4000	NO	YES	50-250	YES	YES	$1750
SynPhonix	NO	YES	ADJUSTABLE	NO	YES	$500
Syntha-Voice	YES	YES	50-700	8K	YES	$600

INTERNAL SPEECH SYSTEMS
===

	Screen Clear	2 Modes: Read/spell	Words/ minute	Buffer	Compatible	Menu	Cost
Accent SA	NO	YES	60-850	8K	YES	NO	$750
Apollo	NO	YES	16 SPEEDS	YES	YES	NO	$1000
Audapter	NO	YES	700	YES	YES	YES	$1100
Personal Speech System	NO	YES (also music)	ADJUSTABLE	2K	YES	NO	$500
Nomad	YES	YES	50-700	8K	YES	NO	$2500
VoxBox	NO	YES	ADJUSTABLE	2K	YES	NO	$700

EXTERNAL SPEECH SYSTEMS

Figure 5. Internal and external speech systems

computer with either a serial or parallel interface. PSS is compatible with several popular software screen readers but not all, so verify that it will work before purchasing. Votrax claims that it will work with a public domain screen reader called "Enable" which would make for a very economical package. Votrax has a contact name and phone number for information about Enable.

VoxBox. VoxBox was developed by InfoBox (Britain) and is distributed by Adhoc Reading Systems. It is garnering a lot of attention because it is economical (depending on the exchange rate under $500), small (weighs only 2-3 pounds), will translate up to seven different languages (only one per unit, however) and has an accuracy rate of 99 percent on industry standard tests. In addition to all of these attributes it also has clear speech due to a "Delta pulse code modulation" technique.

Conclusion

The synthesizer system chosen and the sound quality output is a matter of personal choice and personal budget. There are many who will say that the sounds from DECtalk are the most "human" sounding, while others will say that the words from the SynPhonix card are more accurate. As advised previously, listen to them all and choose the one that will be easiest for your staff to adjust to.

5

Optical Character Recognition (OCR) Systems

Theoretically Optical Character Recognition (OCR) systems, which have the capacity to scan printed text and yield either speech output or to record information to diskette for alternate output (i.e., large print or braille), promise the visually impaired as well as the physically impaired and learning disabled access to the entire print library. In reality, however, the OCRs are not as yet that developed. They will read numerous typefaces, but not all, nor will they read graphics or handwriting (either script or block printing).

Technological advancements of the 90s have brought forth healthy competition to Raymond Kurzweil/Xerox for a piece of the OCR marketplace. Prior to the influx of these new OCRs, persons wanting an OCR had to buy a Kurzweil Reader, which at its "best" occasionally read some print (it was expensive, difficult to use and extremely temperamental) and at its "worst" scared a lot of people from using adaptive technology. However, what the original OCR did was to encourage a major corporation, Xerox, to invest research dollars to enable Kurzweil to perfect his OCR into what is now known as the Xerox/Kurzweil Personal Reader—a superior descendant to the original Kurzweil Reader. The advances Xerox/Kurzweil made also stimulated interest among other companies to research OCR scanning and a competitive market now exists.

Basically, there are three essential elements to OCR technology: scanning (i.e., taking a "picture" of the words), recognition (translating pictures into words), and saving recognized text (or outputting text).[1]

Initially, a printed document is scanned (scanner is similiar to one used in a grocery store, but not the same as commercial scanners which require a large amount of memory) by a camera that contains a photosensitive array. The light and dark images are then sent to a processor where the OCR hardware and software convert these images into recognized characters and the characters into words. The information is then stored in electronic form, either in a PC or a memory buffer of the OCR system (or relayed to the user). The recognition process includes using software algorithms that take into account logical structure of the language (i.e., there is a lexicon, similar to the "spell check" feature of word processors, that automatically corrects the camera mistakes). For instance the camera may see a word "The" at the beginning of a system as "Tke" but will store it correctly, because it checked its lexicon and did not find the word "Tke," but did find that "The" is a word and is commonly used to begin a sentence. All text is saved as temporary files, which are then either read aloud or converted to another usable format.

Popular OCR scanners are currently priced from $3,000-$10,000 as some require a personal computer and some are self-contained. When shopping around for an OCR there are certain items to consider:[2]

1. Can the OCR accurately recognize a wide variety of word processed/typewritten (various font sizes and types including dot matrix) and typeset documents including books, magazines, high-quality print newspapers? (Note: Be sure to use actual material which your intended patron will be using, e.g., if you are intending to use an OCR with the general public who wish to read utility bills and bank statements, include those in the test.)
2. Can the OCR maintain the layout of the original text and recognize columns without user intervention?
3. Does the OCR permit speaking of text as it scans, or permit reading by sentence, paragraph, column, chapter?
4. Can the OCR handle various types of paper sizes (i.e., index card size to legal size)?
5. Does the OCR require a minimum of computer knowledge to operate and come with good documentation and ongoing support from the manufacturer as well as online help functions?
6. Is the scanning process handled at an efficient speed?
7. If the OCR needs to be attached to a PC to function, will it support a variety of PCs?

Three leading OCR readers were tested by the National Technology Center of the American Foundation for the Blind in June 1990 and they will be discussed first. The other scanners discussed are new to the marketplace and will serve as healthy competition to keep prices low and to improve on the product.

Arkenstone Reader

The Arkenstone Reader is a product of Calera Recognition Systems, but is being marketed under the Arkenstone name for a very good reason. Arkenstone is a charitable organization incorporated in 1989 with the sole purpose of "providing technical solutions to charitable needs that are being poorly served by the for-profit or other sectors." Their first major project was to develop an "affordable reading system that really works for the visually or reading impaired." With the cooperation of Calera Recognition Systems (three of the founders sit on the Arkenstone board of directors), the Arkenstone Reader became a reality. This scanner, priced at under $4,000, is distributed through Henter-Joyce as well as forty other distributors of adaptive technology in the U.S. and abroad, as the Reader is capable of reading French and German.

To use the Arkenstone Reader one needs a scanner, a scanner card (card available with purchase) and a PC with adaptive software/hardware (adaptive ware also available with purchase) as well as 4MB of hard drive space. The Arkenstone is relatively easy to use, but like any hardware installation does require someone capable of installing the TrueScan board and loading the software.[3]

Once the hardware and software are in place, the user simply scans the text, presses the space bar on the personal computer and the Arkenstone Reader stores the text in a temporary file and begins to sort through what it sees. It is ready to recall instantly what it has read or store it in a permanent memory file for future recall and possible translation into a special format. Arkenstone was programmed with 1,300 business typefaces in roman, bold and italic, each in sizes varying from 6 to 28 points yielding a total of 16,000 recognizable fonts. It has the ability to read dot-matrix print and has many features such as collating, two-sided page reading and landscape reading. Arkenstone will scan up to 100 characters per second and supports a variety of scanners, including fax boards.

The evaluators at the AFB found that the Arkenstone Reader offered the most features for a PC-based reader.[4] In an article in *PC Magazine* an evaluator claimed that it blew away all other scanners, including the Kurzweil when scanning and reading items such as newsprint and magazine articles and that its only problem lay in the quality of the print not the type.[5] Arkenstone maintains a toll-free technical assistance service for the U.S. and Canada (Pacific Time business hours only).

The PC/KPR

The PC/KPR is a product of Xerox/Kurzweil and is available through Xerox-Kurzweil as well as Celexx, Dotson Enterprises and a host of other independent, licensed dealers. This family of scanners is priced from $4,000-$7,000.

The PC/KPR has not received as much attention as its counterpart the Personal Reader, but nevertheless is as much of an asset to the OCR world as the Personal Reader. It needs to be linked to a personal computer, have a scanner attached and have the scanner card and scanner software installed.

Unlike the Arkenstone Reader, the PC/KPR will work only with the flat-bed scanners provided and a special adapter for a landscape reading is necessary and priced at $1,000. The PC/KPR has the ability to read characters from a point size of 8 to 24 point. The PC/KPR will begin reading the text immediately, rather than storing it to a temporary file, which is a plus for the student not sure if the text in hand will be of value. The reviewers from AFB recommended the PC/KPR for the person wanting only a dedicated read-back machine.[6] There is a toll-free technical assistance line which is staffed by people who actually use the product on a daily basis.

Xerox-Kurzweil Personal Reader (KPR)

The Kurzweil Personal Reader (KPR), a product of Xerox-Kurzweil Industries, is the scanner that has garnered the most attention. This is only partially due to the fact that Xerox has a healthy advertising budget; both Kurzweil and Xerox are known for producing quality and this unit upholds this reputation.

The KPR is available through Celexx Corp., Dotson Industries, and local Xerox-Kurzweil representatives throughout the country and abroad and has a price range of $8,000-$12,000 (depending on scanner option, i.e., hand-held, flatbed, both). Purchase of the unit includes a subscription to the bulletin, "Xerox-Kurzweil Personal Reader Update," and arrangements for special low-cost loans for purchase have been made for individuals and organizations that demonstrate need.[7]

The KPR is a standalone unit that does not require a host PC or the installation of any software; all that is needed to get it scanning and reading is a screwdriver to loosen the scanner from its shipping crate! It comes installed with an enhanced version of DECtalk and an 18-button keypad through which all commands are given to the unit. An optional feature of the KPR is the Infovox synthesizer which will speak in French, German, Spanish, Italian, Swedish, Norwegian and accented British English (one language per card).

The KPR is capable of storing up to 50 pages of scanned printed text at a time and also has the capabilty of reading aloud as the information is being scanned. It also has portability capabilities as the unit, with a hand-held scanner, weighs only 19 pounds and measures 12 1/2 inches by 6 1/2 inches by 17 inches. Users familiar with hand-held scanners may wonder how it is possible for a blind user to scan pages correctly. It is possible through the use of a "magnetic tracking aid" which automatically tracks the text across and down the page.[8]

The KPR already has a following: Larry Scadden, the director of rehabilitation engineering for the Electronic Industries Foundation in Washington, D.C., is impressed by the range of documents the Personal Reader can scan and verbalize. He said that in addition to being able to "read a wide range of documents, technical journals and correspondence it will also accurately read items such as spreadsheets." He went on to say that it can do this because it has the flexibility to "read line-by-line and word-by-word, so each cell is read individually."[9]

The KPR is already a part of quite a few public and state libraries in the United States including the Ridgewood Library of Ridgewood, N.J. The director of this library, when lauding the local Lions club for its donation of a KPR, said "the Kurzweil Personal Reader allows us to extend services to people in our area who are blind, sight-impaired or dyslexic. The size makes it possible to bring the unit to users at home or in schools...we've identified more than eight hundred persons in our area who depend on our services."[10]

The KPR has the advantage of portability as well as the capability of interfacing with a PC, which enables the user to get braille or large-print output as well as the voice. Dr. Fareed Haj, a frequent contributor to *Raised Dots Computing*, sees the KPR as "a means of eradicating illiteracy within the blind or visually impaired community because of the ability to get braille or large print on demand." Dr. Haj is using the KPR to produce items for students in braille (he is transferring the scanner file into the PC, then using the Duxbury translation software), as well as using it to keep up with all his classroom work and leisure reading. The system is not without problems; items such as table of contents, title page, illustrations and footnotes which do not translate properly (i.e., items spaced strangely, punctuation which does not follow rules) will still be a problem. But he contends that it still "is the only way for libraries and schools to provide textbooks in special media."[11]

The next two scanners were not reviewed by the AFB, because of time limitations. New scanners are appearing on the marketplace with regularity.

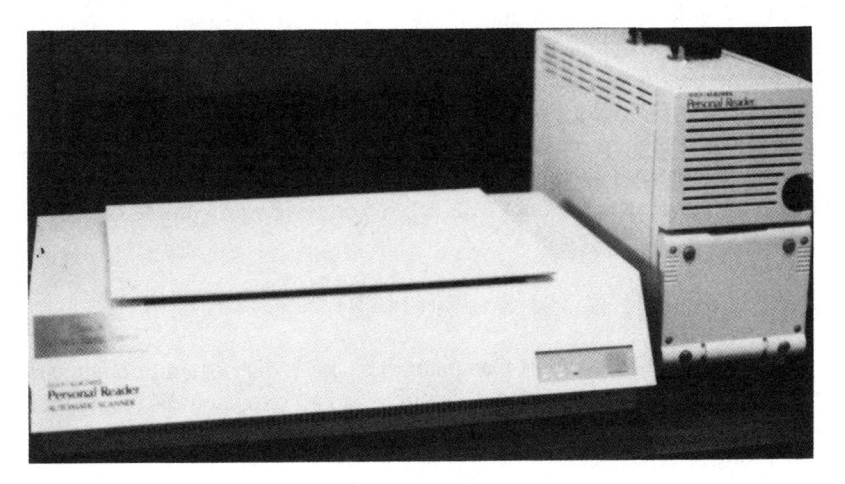

Figure 1. Text scanners have become smaller, less expensive, and easier to use.

An editor of the Sensory Aids Foundation's publication, *Technology Update*, actually summed up the decision-making process of which scanner to buy in the April 1990 issue when he said that the OsCar, Arkenstone and IRIS systems were actually the same and that "what is unique about each is its user interface." There are a few additional subtleties, however, that are worth noting.

OsCar

OsCar was released by TeleSensory in summer 1990 and is priced from $3,900-$4,500. It is essentially the same unit as the Arkenstone Reader in that it used the Calera Recognition system, Truescan. TeleSensory has added one feature—an automatic page orientation analyzer—which could save time. This scanner requires a PC equipped with a speech recognition system. If using other products from TSI (such as a large-print program or embosser), this would be a natural choice. Those who do not have any adaptive equipment may also want to consider OsCar as TSI has several packages available that include OsCar and another type of adaption (e.g., braille translation software) for a discount.

IRIS

IRIS is a product of Visuaide 2000 Inc., of Longueuil, Canada. What makes IRIS unique is that it is a software-only package and allows the user to purchase the recognition card (it is also Calera Truescan) as well as the scanner separately. This piece of software is priced at $395, and takes advantage of the extended keyboard of a standard PC to operate. Reading functions are standard, but also include options such as searching text for words or phrases. The online help feature is also different as it is context-sensitive as well as specific. IRIS also has a simple command to send scanned text to whichever peripheral unit the user desires. The IRIS software will also drive the synthesizer, which means a software driver for the synthesizer would not have to be purchased and as such does not require a screen review program to operate or read text.

ScanRite (ATR)

ScanRite is a product of ATR Computer Tec. and is distributed through various independent representatives. It is priced at approximately $4,600 and requires a PC 286 or 386 with 16-bit internal slot and installed speech synthesizer with software.

	Page orientation	Recognizable font sizes	Versatile typeface	Scanning speed	Reads newsprint	Needs PC interface	Cost
Arkenstone	NO	6-28	YES	75-100 char/sec	YES	YES	$4000-4800
PC/KPR	NO	24	YES	350	NO	YES	$4000-7000
KPR	NO	24	YES	350	NO	NO	$8000-12000
OsCar	YES	6-28	YES	75-100	YES	YES	$3900-4500
ScanRite	NO	6-28	YES	75-100	YES	YES	$46000

Figure 2. Scanners

Once the scanner (flatbed-type) and its software are installed, the typing of a keystroke on a PC will begin the reading process. The unit will recognize typewritten, typeset, laser print, dot-matrix as well as other computer print from 6 to 28 point. There are two models of ScanRite, with the more expensive model being able to recognize up to 100 characters per second (8 seconds per page) and able to create a temporary holding file of up to 50 double-sided pages. The scanner has the ability to handle columns of information effectively. This particular unit has a document feeder similar to that of a laser printer, thus it will hold only letter, legal and government-sized paper.

Summary

Scanners will be making their impact in the world of the visually impaired as well as the learning disabled. Like all technological devices each generation will be more sophisticated and offer the user more for the dollars spent. This current generation does not require a lot of instructional guidance but be aware that, while the personal computer is now familiar to a large segment of the population, the OCR scanners are not.

You should plan for at least one dedicated training session for each user, realizing that there will be some users who will require more than one session. Like clerks who scan books or groceries, some will be good at it and some will not. Once the user is comfortable with the scanning process the mechanics of translating into braille or large print must be reviewed (note: if the user is willing to try the scanning, he or she will probably be computer literate).

6

Keyboards

Software Adaptions for the Keyboard

As mentioned previously, disabilities which prohibit physically handicapped persons from accessing computers are varied. There are some people whose only physical disability is the inability to access more than one side or one key of the computer at a time, which inhibits them from using an application program which calls for the user to press the "CTRL" and "ENTER" keys to define a hard page. For example, the most basic computer application—booting—requires that the user hold down three keys ([CONTROL], [ALT], DEL]) simultaneously, which is impossible for a person lacking manual dexterity without the help of some special software programs which allow the keys to be pressed sequentially and translate them to simultaneous pressing. These software programs also help alleviate key repeats when a key is held down too long by a person who may not be able to move his hands quickly from the keys or may be using a mouth or head stick to push the keys down.[1]

Most of the programs are public domain, although vendors charge a nominal handling fee (under $35) which is used to send future upgrades to registered users as they occur. While there are only slight differences in these programs all of the vendors of these products are willing to send a functional demo disc.

1-KEY

1-KEY is a memory-resident program distributed by Regenesis Development Corp. It was designed to allow the one finger, headstick or mouthstick computer user to use standard software and a standard keyboard (although input may be slow). Depressing and releasing one of the function keys (i.e., SHIFT, CONTROL or ALT) makes it active for the next key allowing the user to sequence his commands. This program also allows the standard key repeat function to be disabled (i.e., only one letter symbol will type regardless of how long the key is held down).

KEYUP

KEYUP, distributed by Ability Systems Corp., allows keys to be pressed sequentially and activates the sequence when the last key is released. It also has a feature that disables the auto repeat feature on standard keyboards but does not have a timed auto repeat feature. It runs transparent to DOS (or any other programs) and occupies less than 3K of memory.

One Finger

One Finger is distributed by the Trace Research Center and allows for "one finger" (or mouthstick or headstick) operation of the SHIFT, CONTROL and ALT keys. The program is "smart" and automatically determines the type of keyboard and computer it is being used with, and can be used with all. It is easy to use—depressing and releasing one of the function keys makes it active turning on or off a program; depressing the key twice locks the key until it is unlocked. The program is memory resident, but can be manually turned off or on. The user can program the automatic repeat of the keys from 0.5 to 60 seconds and to turn itself off.

ENCORE.COM

ENCORE.COM is a shareware software utility of *PC Magazine* and is available directly from *PC Magazine*.[2] While Encore was designed to simply "speed up" repetitive procedures within application programs for the average computer user, when coupled with One Finger or KEYUP it can be a big assist for the computer user who has difficulties making keystrokes. Encore will allow the user to define one keystroke to represent up to 100 keystrokes. A patron who is constantly using one book of a multi-volumed CD-ROM title such as WordCruncher would be able to program one key by typing the command: "CTRL-R: [ret], [ret], 6, 2, CTRL-P", to go directly to the Shakespeare Library, direct look-up, when the user-designated key is pressed again. This program requires 6K of RAM.

Modifications for Standard Keyboards

There are a few adaptions that can be purchased for under $50 that will allow a user with mobility impairments to use the standard computer keyboard. These users need the adaptions for various reasons: one patron may have poor muscle control, while another using a mouthstick may not be able to hit only the key he wants. While these devices will not allow the user to move through searches as quickly as he could with a special keyboard, they will make access less frustrating.

Keyguards

A keyguard is a keyboard overlay with holes positioned over each key. It helps the user to stabilize finger, hand or stick movement and to select a key without accidentally activating others. Keyguards help support the hand and allow the user to slide it across the keyboard without pressing any keys. Keyguards are extremely low cost (approximately $50) and take about a minute to install. They will fit all IBM standard keyboard boards.

Keyguards are available from Prentke-Romich, ComputAbility Corp. and COPH-2. They are all basically the same with a few differences. Prentke-Romich's guard is dark brown and attached with a hook-and-loop device while ComputAbility's is clear and attaches with velcro. The keyguard available from COPH-2 offers a person without firm control of his or her body an economical board which allows him to use a head- or mouthstick to activate only the keys s/he wishes to activate. This control feature is necessary because membrane keyboards are highly sensitive and keys could be activated by the slightest uncontrolled touch.

Key Stoppers

KeyStoppers, a trademark of Hoolean, are different from keyguards in that they will disable specific keys that are deemed "hazardous" to the user who can use a standard keyboard, but needs to be safeguarded from accidently hitting keys like "EXIT" or "DELETE" through involuntary body motions. There are two types of KeyStoppers: "soft" and "hard." The soft KeyStopper will partially immobilize the key and require the user to exert more pressure to use it. The hard KeyStopper will prevent operation of the key altogether. These kits are easy to use—simply remove the keys with the key pulling device supplied, insert the soft or hard KeyStopper over the slot the key stem inserts into, then replace the key, pushing firmly until it clicks. The cost for a kit of four hard and four soft KeyStoppers as well as the key puller is under $15.00 including shipping.

Key locking devices should also be available through your PC manufacturer and are available from Hoolean and L S & S Group without any notations on them.

Disk Guides

While not part of the keyboards, disk guides allow the computer user with poor hand control to access computers more easily. The disk guide is positioned on a stable surface (unlike the "mid-way" up position of the "A" or "B" drives on most computers) allowing the user to steady his hand on the surface as he aligns the diskette with the drive opening. The guide attaches as easily as any added drives and is available as a replacement to both internal drives and external drives.

The disk guide is priced at approximately $100 and available through Prentke-Romich and TASH as well as other distributors offering basic adaptive computer devices.

Keyboards

Several different types of keyboards are currently available which enable the user with limited hand or wrist movement to access the computer for information. Typically these patrons would be able to read the screen or listen to a screen reader, but for some reason (arthritis, cerebral palsy, neurological damage) cannot physically type commands on a standard keyboard. They may lack the coordination to give commands requiring the user to hold down three keys at a time (ex. DOS boot command of ALT-CONTROL-DEL) or lack the ability to expand their hand to type keys using the typical five-row spread of a typical keyboard. For some patrons the problem is as major as lacking the strength and or coordination skills to physically depress any key for the computer to receive the signal that this is the key the user wants.[3] There are simple ways to solve the keyboard access problem and most are easily installed, low cost (under $1,000) and will not cause the non-impaired user problems if used as the keyboard for a shared terminal. Most of these keyboards also allow for reconfiguration of keys to allow the user to use his/her physical ability to the maximum. Figure 1 illustrates some typical reconfigurations.

Membrane Keyboards

Membrane keyboards would assist patrons who do not have the physical ability to depress individual keys on a standard keyboard and would also be of help to the visually impaired person who needs a larger typeface key than commercial large-print keytops provide. The keys require various degrees of downward pressure to activate. There are some that will activate with half an ounce of pressure for persons who have coordination but lack strength to activate as well as keyboards requiring almost a pound of downward pressure for those who have strength but lack coordination (a key on a standard keyboard could be activated with about 2 oz. of downward pressure). These keyboards make it possible for a person able to hold a stick with some body part (i.e., mouth, little finger) to manipulate that stick to punch out commands and use the resources found on the computer without accidently activating unwanted keys. These keyboards are similar to keypads found on

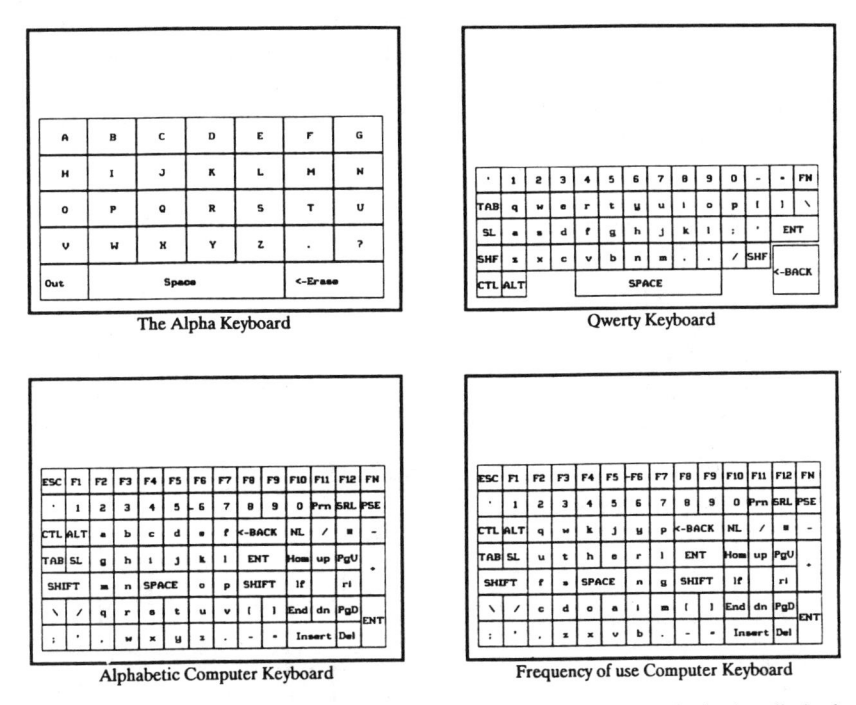

Figure 1. The ability to reprogram computer keys aids the individual who has limited mobility. Source: "Eyegaze Computer System for the Physically Handicapped," LC Technologies, Inc., 1989.

some pocket calculators (i.e., flat with surface notations) and have a "high-tech" design thus could serve as the keyboard in a shared disabled/abled workstation.

The membrane keyboards come in two sizes: "expanded" with large squares replacing keys and "small" with pocket-calculator-sized keys replacing the standard keyboard keys. The keyboard size chosen depends on needs of the user; an expanded keyboard would be needed by the individual who can target only large areas and the miniature keyboards would be used by those with an extremely limited range of movement of their limbs.

Most of the keyboards allow the user to reprogram the keyboard (overlays provided for re-lettering prompts) to make the most use of the physical strength or mobility available (i.e., standard keyboard layout not the most logical in relation to usage). Those that enable the user to reconfigure the board need a hardware adapter or interface card, which will translate user commands for the computer. The most used interface cards are AID + ME, PC Serial AID and Breakthru Box.

76 Library Technology for Visually and Physically Impaired Patrons

While there are not as many manufacturers of these specialized keyboards (compared to a standard keyboard), there are enough to make purchase of one possible for under $1,000, including the interface. Figure 2 is representative of an actual, large-membrane keyboard, assigned the QWERTY configuration.

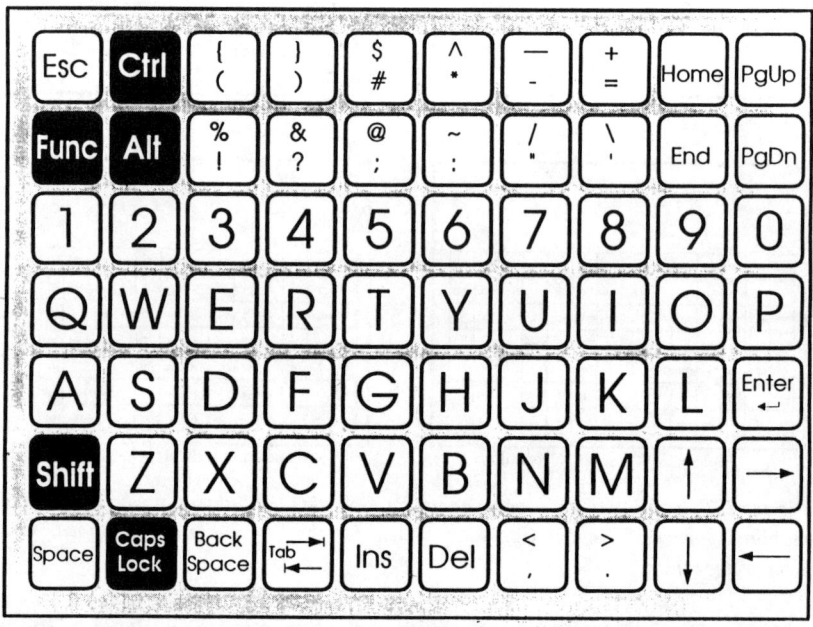

Figure 2. This is an actual reproduction of an expanded membrane keyboard.

Larger Keyboards

EKEG Expanded Keyboard. The EKEG Expanded Keyboard is a product of EKEG Electronics, Ltd. of British Columbia, Canada and is priced at $750. It is presently sold by the manufacturer, TASH and Prentke-Romich. It was designed to operate exactly like an IBM keyboard, with the only difference being that its keys are 1.5" square and the board is perfectly flat, and the keys require about 15 ounces of downward pressure to activate. This keyboard is equipped with firmware which allows a "latching" device (i.e., permits the user to hold down function keys like the DOS boot commands key until he is able to press down the next key needed) to exist. This keyboard is also equipped with a microprocessor which allows an adjustable delay to accept a key (e.g., Shift Key and the F8 key) sequence. Additionally there is an adapter available ($75) that will allow a standard keyboard to remain in place if desired. Another feature of the EKEG keyboard is that a keyguard is available for $50 that will exactly fit over this keyboard.

Expanded Membrane Keyboard and Keyboard II. The Expanded Membrane Keyboard and Membrane Keyboard II are products of Comput-Ability Corporation. These low-cost keyboards ($200-$300 respectively) require an adaptive interface card (will use card from AID+ME, ComputAbility; PC Serial Aid, Don Johnston Developmental Equipment; Adaptive Firmware Card, LS &S, TASH) which is inserted into a slot in the computer. These keyboards, which require almost a pound of downward pressure to activate, are not as sensitive as standard keyboards which is good for persons with poor dexterity or spastic muscles causing them to regularly strike unwanted keys.

The key space for each of the 128 programmable keys on the Expanded Membrane Keyboard measures 1.25" square and possesses an active area size of 20" x 10". In addition to allowing redefinition of key combinations (each key can take up an area of 4" if needed), unique features allow the Expanded Membrane Keyboard to emulate mouse cursor control, which can be controlled by a keystroke or a mouse button. The keys do require a force of 15 ounces to activate, meaning that the individual using the keyboard must press down with force.

The Membrane Keyboard II is programmable (i.e., allows reassignment of keys) and requires a 15-ounce force to activate the 128 keys. It measures approximately 13" x 7" and, unlike the Expanded Membrane Keyboard, it will not emulate mouse movement. The "non-mouse" emulation would be significant if you planned to develop a system that would take advantage of programs that demand the use of a mouse.

Keyport 300

Keyport 300 is a product of Polytel Computer Products and has a feature that sets it apart from other keyboards—the number of key options and the layout of these keys. Like its name indicates, there are 300 programmable keys (or combinations) arranged in 20 rows and 15 columns (approximately 8 1/2" x 11"). Each key is 1/2" square and gives the user a one-touch access to a program's command sequence or a series of keystrokes needed to work through menus. Common letter combinations (e.g., "er", "is", "and"), common words (e.g., the, and, but) and even commonly used phrases (e.g., Thank you for your interest) can be programmed, allowing the user to input information more quickly by touching one key. While this is a boon to the disabled keyboard users, the non-disabled might also find it of value.

Programming keys is a straightforward procedure: the user would start the program by typing "KPSTART," "SET NEW," and then issue the definitions. For example a user who may want to access a CD-ROM title may define Key 1 to make the keyboard "type" the log-on process (ex.: Type CD\ee [ret] wait, Type ee); use Key 2 to choose one type of access route he or she wants to take (ex.: for Word Search, Type [enter], [enter]") and use Key 3 for his or her exit route from the program (e.g.: type [ALT Q], wait, type "enter"). The user would then type "KPEND" to save these commands. There is even a simpler programming version called "on-the-fly" programming, whereby the user would press the "ALT" key and then the key he wished to define, then the keystroke sequence and then the "ALT" key and the defined key again. This programming version would work only if the user could hold down two keys simultaneously. In the case of a shared terminal, all keyboard definitions can be saved on a diskette for future use.

It should be noted that although Keyport was not specifically designed for the disabled (but rather for the restaurant business to aid order takers in quickly inputting food requests), its low price of $250 (which includes an interface that allows it to work at the same time as a standard keyboard) makes it a very tempting choice among the membrane keyboards; its drawback is the small key size and the need to exert some pressure to activate the keys.

Keyport 176

This keyboard has all the features of the Keyport 300, but has larger keys, (5/8") as well as tactile feedback; there is a raised "bubble" on each key area which would be of help to orient the visually impaired user. The overall keyboard size is 8 1/2" x 11" which makes it possible to use standard paper to create a written record of the defined keyboard layout (plastic overlays provided) for multiple users and their definitions. This Polytel product is priced for commercial use (under $200) and can serve as an economical keyboard access. The drawbacks are that even though the keys are larger on the Keyport 176 than the 300 model they are still relatively small for an alternate input keyboard and require a firm downward pressure to activate, making it difficult for a person with poor muscle control or visual impairment to use.

The Unicorn Expanded Keyboard II

Available from L S & S Group, TASH and Prentke-Romich, the Unicorn Expanded Keyboard II has become a standard in the adaptive technology field. It has 128 large (1-1/4") user-definable keys, which can be grouped together as needed to form combinations such as "ALT-CONTROL-DEL"; these keys require the capability of exerting 6 oz. of downward pressure to activate. The large-sized spaces are for the user who either has a visual disability or a coordination disability (there is a large target area). The selected keyboard can be changed simply for each user by storing the chosen layout on diskette. Unicorn recognized the fact that the PC will be accessed by a variety of users with different needs (i.e., one user may be able to use a few fingers on her right hand, while another user may be using a mouthstick) and provides overlays that can be written on and saved for each individual user. The inputting of the keyboard selection is easy for the novice as helpful prompts walk you through the keyboard selection.

The keyboard is priced at $350, but requires PC Serial AID (can run on either COM1 or COM2) priced at $400 to facilitate the recognition of the keyboard by the PC. This allows one to redefine the keyboard to user needs as well as allow for mouse emulation and access to all IBM codes. Additionally this accessory will enable a user to enter input using Morse code and have it translated to ASCII, which is used for severely mobility-limited individuals who must tap out their messages using a Morse Code Key.

Should you determine that your patrons need the ability to enter data using a membrane keyboard, but don't necessarily need the ability to rearrange the keyboard, a model of the same keyboard is available which will plug directly into the keyboard jack and needs no special adaptions. This is priced at approximately $750, and has the ability to attach and detach quickly.

Smaller-Sized Keyboards

Bloorview Miniature Keyboard. Introduced in 1990, the Bloorview Miniature Keyboard was developed by Bloorview Childrens Hospital in Toronto, Canada and is being distributed by TASH and Bloorview Hospital. The Bloorview Miniature Keyboard uses an actual Sharp 1360 pocket computer (the type used by various manufacturers for dictionaries, notepads, etc.) and a custom cable. The Sharp computer runs a software program to allow all keystrokes of the regular keyboard to be typed from the Sharp and connects directly into the keyboard port of the PC. Additionally, the Bloorview Keyboard allows the standard keyboard to remain in place, if a port can be adapted.

The Bloorview is extremely sensitive, and requires only 1 oz. of downward pressure to activate. The Bloorview is able to emulate a standard keyboard through the use of the "Mode" feature, which when activated will turn an alpha key into a TAB key. This keyboard is ideal for any user who has limited but precise movement, such as a child with arthritic hands

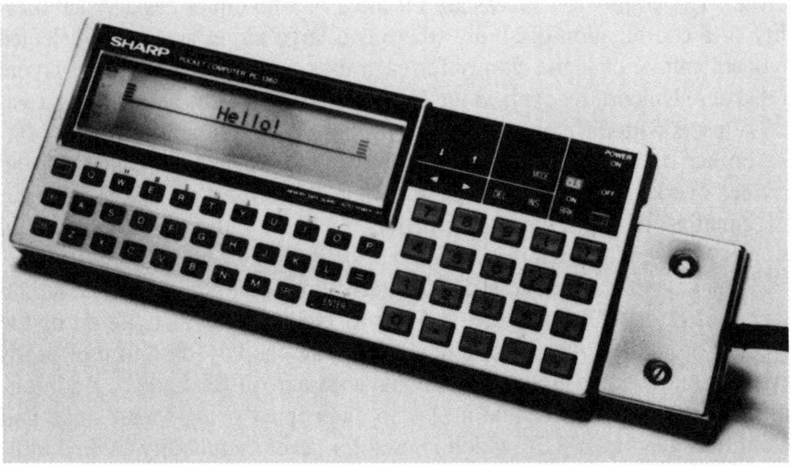

Figure 3. The Bloorview keyboard fits in the palm of an adult's hand yet has all the functions of a standard keyboard. The smaller keyboard makes "reaching" for keys easier for some individuals. Photo courtesy of TASH.

Keyport 60. Keyport 60, priced at under $125, is manufactured and distributed by Polytel Computer Products. It is a unique membrane keyboard in that it was designed to work with a standard keyboard in place. It is 12" x 2.5" x .25" and is designed to be affixed to the top part of a standard IBM keyboard with adhesive pads (although not necessary) and plugs into the game port of the PC. Keys, which require over an ounce of downward pressure to activate, are arranged in three rows of 20 and allow the user to assign and reassign up to 60 key combinations when needed by using a feature of the supplied software that transfers each pattern used to diskette for future use. This feature is extremely useful if working with various types of software having different function commands (i.e., SHIFT, PG DN or TAB, DOWN ARROW) to retrieve information or browse data.

Mini Keyboard. Mini Keyboard is a product of ComputAbility Corporation, which markets and distributes them. It is priced at approximately $150. It does require an interface card and while the company's own product, AID+ME, is recommended, it will also work with: Serial Aid (available from Don Johnston Developmental Equipment) and the Adaptive Firmware Card (available from L S & S and TASH).

While it is not as sensitive as some keyboards, it will activate when 1.5 ounces of force is applied. There are 70 keys which are user definable. The board is only 7" x 5" and weighs approximately one pound.

PC Mini Keyboard. PC Mini Keyboard is a product of TASH Inc., is priced at $700 and can be plugged directly into the keyboard port without requiring any additional hardware or software. The Tash PC Mini Keyboard requires a force of 3.5 ounces to activate keys which means they can be activated with a mouthstick, pointer or fingers and allows the user to set response time from 0 to 2 seconds which allows the user with a slow response time to linger on a key without it repeating. This keyboard also has an audio feedback feature which indicates when a key is pressed and when the information is sent to the computer, again helpful to the user who may not know if pressure applied to a key was sufficient to activate a computer response. The keyboard also has a simultaneous "lighted latching" (e.g., CTRL, ALT, SHIFT and other Functions) feature, which alerts the user to the functions being on or off.

TASH also sells the same keyboard requiring an adaptive firmware card to operate for $360.

The Unicorn Mini Keyboard. The Unicorn Mini Keyboard is based on the same engineering principles as the Unicorn Expanded Keyboard. The Mini is designed for individuals with limited hand expansion or body movement (with coordination) who wish to access the personal computer. It requires the individual to exert only 3 ozs. of downward pressure to activate the keys. Like the Expanded Keyboard, the Mini can be reprogrammed to move frequently used keys or key-groupings to suit the user needs. This keyboard measures 7 1/2" x 4 1/2" x 1/2" (basically the size of an adult hand). The Unicorn Mini, is priced at $250 and requires the PC Serial AID and the ability to connect to the COM1 or COM2 port.

There is also a "quick install" version of the Mini Keyboard available at a cost of $700 for those who do not need the option to reconfigure the keyboard. Like the Expanded Keyboard II, the Mini will plug directly into the keyboard jack, without any other type of installation needed.

	# of keys	Sentence programmable	Size	Overlays	Interface needed	Type of interface	Type (Expander/Small)	Cost
Keyport 300	300	YES	1/2"	YES	YES	GAMEPORT	E	$240
Keyport 176	176	YES	5/8"	YES	YES	GAMEPORT	E o	$200
Unicorn	128	NO	1.25"	YES	YES	SERIAL	E	$385
Bloorview	61	NO	<1/4"	NO	NO	N/A	S	CALL
Keyport 60	60	NO	1/4"	NO	YES	GAMEPORT	S	$125
Mini Keyboard	70	NO	1/4"	NO	YES	AID+ME	S	$150
PC Mini Keyboard	64	NO	1/4"	NO	NO	N/A	S	$700

Figure 4. Keyboards

Summary

Specialized keyboards can be useful to the "able-bodied" as well as needed by the disabled. The keyboards are all easy to use, and also function as a standard keyboard, meaning the $1,000 (or less) investment will always be used.

7

Processing Information Without a Keyboard

Limited mobility device is a term used to describe the devices and applications which assist persons who cannot physically input information into a computer because of physical limitations. This diverse grouping of devices allows persons with the most minimal of voluntary control (even the usage of an eye muscle is sufficient) to access the computer and be part of the information exchange. Some of these devices are highly specialized and will be of use to extremely small populations of persons with specific and varying degrees of disability. While it is not feasible to purchase every conceivable type of alternative input device you should be aware of the items that are available and strive to acquire them as needed.

Before beginning a discussion of these elite computer adaptions for physically impaired information seekers it is necessary to discuss one basic need: furniture designed for the physically handicapped. Keep in mind that patrons using a wheelchair to navigate the library and access the computer have to be able to "wheel" themselves under the table on which the computer rests; choose furniture which will allow this. Also be sure that the computer is at a comfortable viewing height; persons in wheelchairs spend a lot of their time "looking up" and anything that can be done to alleviate this is a plus. There is a lot of computer furniture in the marketplace that is suitable for wheelchair access. And there are companies like CLEO, Inc., ComputAbility, Prentke-Romich and ZYGO that sell or will custom design a workstation for your library's needs. They include stations that are height adjustable and have tilt-down keyboard trays which allow the user ease in typing.[1]

Darci Joystick

Anyone who has played a computer game has used a joystick and will recognize DARCI as a joystick rather than a true keyboard. DARCI is manufactured by WesTest Engineering and priced at just under $1,000. It is so sophisticated that this "joystick" can be used in place of a keyboard or alongside a standard keyboard. DARCI has been preprogrammed to respond to eight possible positions, with each pattern representing a single character, word or command. DARCI works in four modes of operation—letter, word, number and cursor control—which means the user can use DARCI to enter information a letter at a time or a word at a time, increasing user possibilities. DARCI also has a latching mode which will allow function keys to be locked together for DOS commands or specific program commands. DARCI's movements are easy to learn and DARCI is easy to install inasmuch as it plugs directly into the keyboard port and does not require an interface. DARCI is used by individuals who can control a joystick, but not key movements.

Mouse Entry

While there exist software programs that call for a mouse to take them through various menus, there are people who use a mouse to input all of their information into the computer. These users are able to grasp a mouse either with their hand or foot and roll it and click its keys until their messages are input into the computer. There are several types of mice available which are designed to help people with certain types of disabilities overcome them and access information.

PowerMouse 100

One such mouse is actually a combination mouse and programmable keypad.[2] This device, called PowerMouse100, is a product of ProHance Technologies. It was not designed specifically for the disabled user, thus it is reasonably priced at under $300. In addition to a low price tag, an interface card is not a requirement. It has 40 programmable keys that allow the user to program each with a command string of up to 255 keystrokes. Additionally, these 40 keys can be linked together to produce 240 macros, giving the user freedom from repetitious but needed strokes. The drawback of PowerMouse 100 is that it works with its own device driver and will not work with MicroSoft Windows, which limits its uses as many software programs are driven by MicroSoft's Windows.[3]

PC-TRAC

A product of MicroSpeed, Inc., PC-TRAC emulates a mouse, but does not actually have to be moved. It has three buttons on it which when depressed will start the cursor moving, a motion device driver monitors the rate at which the cursor is moved and adjusts the speed from 50-1000 pulses per inch. This allows the person unable to lift his or her finger off the mouse button quickly to take his or her time, as the cursor is moving at operators speed not the standard keyboard speed. PC-TRAC is budget priced at under $150.

Mouse-Trak

Mouse-Trak is made by Itac Systems and is actually a 2" trackball that allows the user to rest his wrist on a cushioned pad while the fingers activate the two or three programmable buttons positioned at the end of the pad. The buttons are programmable to facilitate its use in various programs. For instance, the buttons may be programmed to emulate the space bar and down/up arrows for one CD-ROM title and may be programmed as the space bar and left/right arrow for another. Mouse-Trak is easy to use as it connects directly into the mouse port and does not interfere with the keyboard functions.

Footmouse

Footmouse is a product of Versatron Corporation and is sold basically at cost ($50). The Footmouse controls cursor movements and allows the user to have the freedom to move the cursor anywhere he wants it to be. The base of the Footmouse remains on the floor, and the cursor is moved by sliding the foot over the base in an up, down, left, right motion and even emulates the auto-repeat feature found on standard keyboards. Footmouse is extremely easy to install, as it plugs directly between the keyboard and the computer. It does not interfere with the usage of the standard keyboard.

The Interface Card/Hardware and Software

As noted in some of the descriptions of the membrane keyboards (others had this built into the keyboard), firmware adapter interface cards are needed to alert the computer to the fact that the input it will receive will not be the traditional type it was programmed to receive. There are several interface devices that allow the user to input information using the membrane keyboards as well as scanning, Morse code entry, touch windows and sip or puff switches.

AID + ME

A product of ComputAbility, AID + ME, priced at $750, allows standard software to be run using a variety of alternative input devices. AID + ME is programmed to work with 16 alternate keyboards, switches and other input devices (it allows other input devices to be programmed for its use). It has an internal speech synthesizer which is a plus for the visually impaired user and is connected to the serial interface and keyboard (if mouse emulation is needed it can also be attached to mouse port).

PC Serial AID

PC Serial AID is a product of Don Johnston Developmental Equipment Inc. It is approximately $400 and is available from TASH, L S & S as well as Johnston. PC Serial AID can be plugged directly into the serial port (PC AID plugs into the parallel port) and will allow functions like scanning, single/dual switch Morse code and keyboard redefinition to be accessed. The interface runs transparently with most programs and gives verbal output.

Breakthru Box

Breakthru Box is a product of EKEG Electronics Ltd., and is priced under $500. This product is literally a "smart" electronics box which plugs into the keyboard socket of the computer and the keyboard (or adaptive data entry device) and allows the user to immediately access items such as the membrane keyboards. The Breakthru Box is said to work with most of the commercially available adaptive keyboard entry programs, but it should be noted that the electronics in the box are all EKEG meaning that the keyboard should be EKEG-compatible. An added feature to the Breakthru Box makes it unique; it has a dip switch which allows for repeat characters (i.e., if a user constantly is typing ***, the switch can be set to repeat three times when pressed once).

CINTEX

While not a hardware or firmware device, CINTEX is a software product of NanoPac which also serves as the interface between the personal computer and a variety of adaptive input contact switches (eyebrow, sip and puff), keyboards or joysticks. The basic package is expensive ($1,150), but incredible. It is a word processor that has the "sticky key" feature (i.e., grouping of the function keys), has word prediction ability (i.e., will learn words used most frequently and type them in, saving the user time) and musical composition abilities. For additional dollars it can also have the ability to control the environment (for instance the user can access the computer for information and also turn on a VCR which has a video tutor program on it or dial a help-line number for the patron who cannot physically do these things himself).

CINTEX will work with almost all alternate input methods, including voice commands. It requires a lot of memory; a full 640K. This means that CINTEX and DOS could not function together in most PC memories without modifications. These modifications are not difficult, but it may mean establishing special boot procedures for each program needed to be run. Once established, these procedures would be straightforward and stored on diskette for the users.

DADA Entry

DADA Entry was introduced in 1990 by Designing Aids for Disabled Adults. The hardware of this device is a mere 4" x 6" x 1" but it has powerful software which enables it to act as the translator of alternate input devices such as switch-activated scanners, 1, 2 or 3 switch Morse Code, as well as virtually all alternate keyboards. The software has a feature which completes words for users (using word prediction) who are inputting messages through a tedious process such as head scanning or Morse code. An abbreviation feature allows a user to develop and store a lexicon of words he commonly uses along with the abbreviation he will be using so that when he types the abbreviation the word or sentence will be recalled and entered into the working document.

The abbreviation feature is a menu-driven procedure which is not difficult to use. If the user finds that there is a word or phrase that he is constantly using (e.g., "Sincerely Yours," in letter writing), he would add it to his dictionary when he types the phrase by:

1. choosing options <S>-Save current Directory from the Word Completion Dictionary (entered by typing: <alt><W>);
2. choose the dictionary that he will turn on whenever he formats a letter, ex. <let>;
3. press <return>.

Now, each time the user writes a letter in this dictionary and starts to type "Si" the words "Sincerely Yours" will appear, saving time and keystrokes. This product has received positive review from TASH in its July 1990 *Update* Newsletter and is available for purchase for $900 from either DADA or L S & S.

	Windows	Speech	Mouse	Joystick	Membrane keyboards	Switch by scanning	Type (Hard/Soft)	Word Prediction	Cost
AID+ME	YES	YES	YES	YES	YES	YES	H	NO	$750
Breakthru BX	NO	NO	NO	NO	YES (large only)	NO	H	NO	$475
PC Serial AID	NO	YES	NO	NO	YES	YES	H	NO	$700
DADA Entry	YES	YES	YES	YES	YES	YES	S	YES	$900
CINTEX	YES	YES	YES	YES	YES	YES	S	YES	$700

Figure 1. Interfaces for adaptive devices

Switches

Compared to previously discussed alternate methods of inputting information into the computer by persons unable to access the standard keyboard, switches are probably the most radically different format. Switches are used only by the most severely physically disabled. Switches, when used in conjunction with hardware or software devices, provide input to the computer identical to typing in the information using a conventional keyboard. The device works as a transcriber, and translates or "switches" the input language of the user to keyboard language which the computer recognizes.

As seen in Figure 2, a wide variety of switches are activated by almost any voluntary motion of the body. This means that a quadriplegic may still use a computer because he can move his head or raise an eyebrow or puff on a tube. The power of switches is so great that not only can a computer be run with them, but entire home and library environments can be controlled by a computer with switch interfaces! These configurations are liberating many a brilliant mind, allowing them independence and intellectual growth.

Because there is such a wide variety of switches available, there are "needs assessment" professionals at: Prentke-Romich, TASH, ComputAbility, ZYGO and DU-IT who are able to determine the right type of switch to be used by the impaired individual by conducting a battery of tests. It is highly unlikely that one specific switching configuration will be used by more than one person using your library. In fact, the reason that there are so many types of switching devices available today is because some severely physically impaired individual somewhere needed an entry point to communication and someone capable of designing it did so and made it available to others.[4] The person using switches may know what switch he can use and bring the switching device with him if he knows that the library will provide a computer with an adaptive serial interface, a port(s) and software which can be used with his switch. Should the individual not know which switch would help him the most, it is advisable to contact one of the previously mentioned companies and at least discuss, however superficially, what could be done for this person.[5]

While it is impossible to purchase switches in anticipation of need, an interface card or software purchased and installed in the computer will allow access and growth of switch applications. Most are highly versatile and capable of multiple functions (i.e., will serve as the interface for a membrane keyboard and a switch). Should you find a switch user constantly bringing one of his own devices with him on library visits, you can purchase one for use in the library as they are all inexpensive ($100-$250). The following discussion is provided to orient the reader to the possible solutions to computer access difficulties caused by severe physical handicaps. There are some instances when a combination of these switches will be needed and used to gain access.[6]

Mouth Control Using Sip and Puff Switches

Puff and Sip switches serve as the vehicle to emulate the physical action of using the keyboard keys and joysticks. For the individual who does not have constant control of his hands and cannot depress a key there are puff and sip switches available. Pressure (puffing) and suction (sipping) through disposable straws dictates the direction in which the cursor will move. These switches can be used to activate several computer applications such as an on-screen keyboard or Morse code. The individual moves the cursor by puffing until it reaches the key s/he wants to input and then sipping to tell the computer that this letter is the desired choice. There are varying degrees of pressure needed to activate the devices, but all need some type of interface (either hardware or software) to alert the computer to look for the "sips" and "puffs" and recognize them as keyboard functions. All of the switches need a software program to serve as the access medium which takes the place of the keyboard. The sampling discussed here is just that—a sampling. There are at least a dozen different puff and sip switches available, designed to meet the individuals' abilities and needs.

4-Pneumatic Switch. The 4-Pneumatic Switch is a product of ZYGO Industries and is a switching unit that accepts input from a sip and puff tube. Since it has four switches, combinations of sips and puffs are used to activate each of them. This switch can be used to choose letters from a screen keyboard or input letters via Morse code (appropriate application software is needed). This switch is also available as a dual control which can connect to a variety of secondary switches or devices. This same switch is also offered from Prentke-Romich, TASH and DU-IT under a slightly different name.

Air Cushion Switch (Single and Dual)

The Air Cushion Switch is a product of Prentke-Romich, ComputAbility and TASH. It consists of an air bellows with a tube leading to the switching unit which translates the signal into ASCII and sends it to the computer. By lightly puffing on the air bellows, air pressure is sent to the switching unit where the change in pressure activates the switch and the computer gets the signal that a command is being given. These units have the capability of activating one or two sets of bellows for single or dual switching.

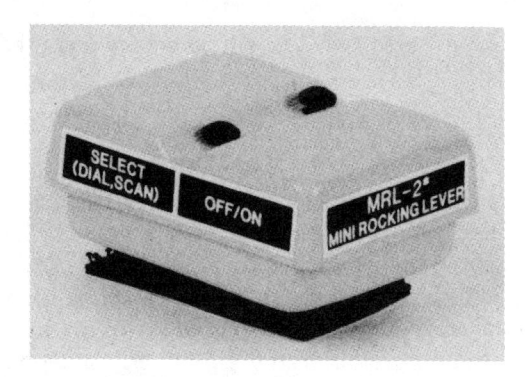

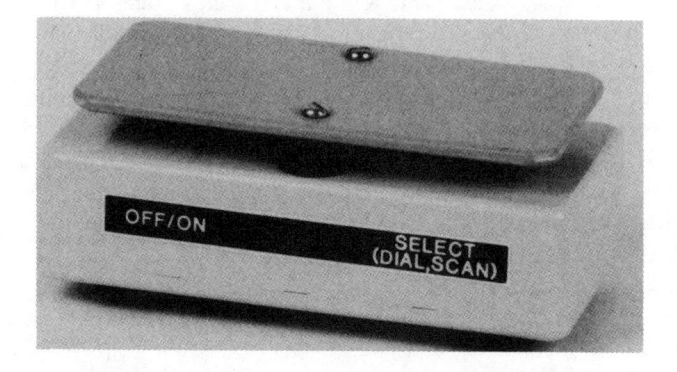

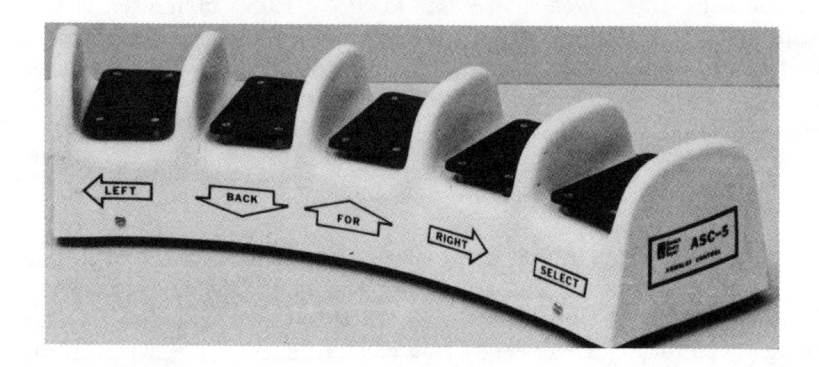

90 Library Technology for Visually and Physically Impaired Patrons

Figure 2. Various switches make it possible for virtually all users to access technology and life. From top to bottom: Mini Rocking Lever Switch, courtesy Prentke-Romich; Dual Switch, courtesy Prentke-Romich; Armslot Switch Controller, courtesy DU-IT Control Systems.

Processing Information Without a Keyboard 91

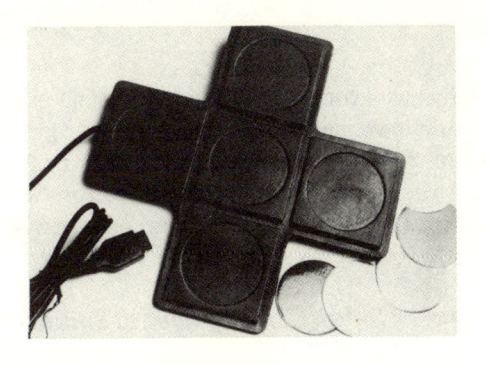

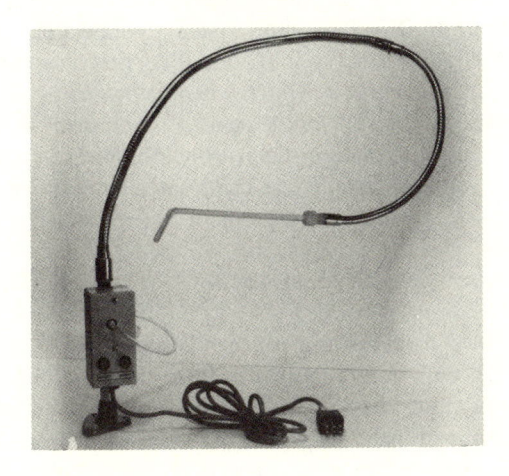

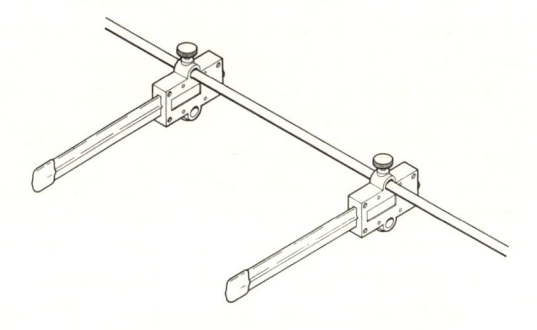

Figure 2 (cont). *From top to bottom: Star, courtesy TASH Inc.; Puff-Sip Dual Switch, courtesy DU-IT Control Systems; LEAF, courtesy ZYGO Industries, Inc.*

Arm Control

For the individual with control of his arm, switching units controlled by slight (but definite) arm movements can allow access to computers. The individual's arm rests in a cradle of slots, each with its own switch; as the arm is moved from switch to switch the computer gets the user's input message. They also need a software program such as Morse code or a screen keyboard to serve as a keyboard.

Arm Slot Control/Armslot Switch Control/5-Thread Switch Slot Control

Arm Slot Control is a product of Prentke-Romich, Armslot Switch Control is a product of DU-IT Control Systems Group, Inc. and 5-Thread Switch Slot Control is a product of ZYGO. All devices have a series of five switches arranged in a semi-circle, which when depressed by arm movement will input information. The slots are separated by dividers to eliminate the possibility of accidental activation. Each switch controls a possible cursor movement (i.e., forward, backward, left, right, select) and activation of one is equivalent to key pressure or mouse movement.

Finger Control/Hand Control/Wrist Control

The variation on hand and finger usage is something most of us do not think about; we just do it and do not realize that there are different motions involved in pressing a key downward or flipping a rocker switch. For some individuals, variations on hand usage are very important as these variations and adaptions help them communicate. For some users, their most controlled input may be done with one finger. These individuals cannot use a miniature keyboard with keys because they cannot move their hand in a controlled manner or extend their finger and press downward on a key. However, by slipping their finger into a secured switching chamber they can raise their finger up and down to tap out a code which will translate into keystrokes. Others may be able to move their finger slightly to the left or right and "rock" out messages using a rocker switch. These switches also work in conjunction with a software package emulating a keyboard (usually a screen keyboard).

There are several types of button switches that can be activated by a simple downward pressure. These switches are manufactured principally by ZYGO, DU-IT Control Systems, Crestwood, TASH, Prentke-Romich and Don Johnston. They operate basically the same way, with the differences being the amount of pressure needed to activate, configuration and number of buttons which translates to the number of switches.

ZYGO and TASH both manufacture a 4-Pushbutton Switch and a 5-Pushbutton Switch which is a set of four/five snap-action buttons switches housed side-by-side on a pad (respectively called 4 or 5 Pushbutton Switch and Penta Switch). Each button, which resembles a doorbell button, gives a movement command such as left or right which translate into keyboard right or left commands.

ZYGO manufactures a Thumb switch which allows the person who has control of only his thumb to input commands to the computer. The device resembles a combination of a "nurse call switch" and a "thumb brace." The "brace," steadies the thumb to allow for precise movements and sends them to the "nurse call switch" which in turn sends the commands to the computer.

DU-IT Control Systems, Don Johnston and Prentke-Romich also make buttons that can be mounted in a manner that allows for activation when touched which a deliberate force by any body part. Again, there are variations on control with computer users with severe mobility limitations and again there are answers. For the user who cannot hone in on a button as small as a doorbell there exists the alternative of plates, which are larger and more sensitive (many are made of the same combination of plastic and electronics found in the membrane keyboards). These plate switches are distributed by ZYGO, Don Johnston, TASH and Prentke-Romich. They can be housed side-by-side as in the ZYGO model or as a star design in the TASH design; the model selected should be the one which is activated by the voluntary motion most often duplicated by the user.

If a user can more easily activate a large rocker switch because it involves a "flipping" motion toward a large target area, rather than a downward motion, then there are several rocker switching units available. These units are made by Prentke-Romich (Dual Rocking Lever Switch and Mini Rocking Lever Switch), Don Johnston (Left/Right Rocker Switch) and TASH (Rocker Switch) and are available in various activation models (low to high force). They will activate two switches and give the user at least two signaling possibilities.

For the user who cannot push either a button, plate or rocker switch there is a unique switch called the String Switch. This switch is manufactured by Ablenet, and is literally activated by the lifting of a string. This quite naturally is a slow input process, but nevertheless allows the mind to work, communicate and learn. Other users may only have control of their wrists but are able to coordinate their wrist and make it push the hand ever so lightly and make contact with switches called leafs and levers. Leaf switches are round and mounted on a T-bar unit at a height the user can easily interact with. This unit requires only a simple push to activate the signal switch (1/4" in one direction) and can actually work with any controlled body part. Levers are akin to a "see-saw"; lightly pressing one side will cause movement in one direction and activate one switch while pressing the other side of the lever will cause a different switch to activate. Leaf- and lever-type switches are available from TASH and ZYGO Industries.

Some persons may have the ability to grasp a small joystick and as a result are able to make use of the joystick's possible four positions to input information and to command the computer. Inputting is much easier with a joystick than with buttons or plates, because joysticks are a recognized input device in the standardized computer world. These joysticks resemble a standard joystick used for games, but either are a lot smaller or do not require as much pressure to activate. The joystick must work with a software program such as a screen keyboard. The joystick allows the user to move from key to key on screen with the up/down and left/right movements and select the key he wishes with another device.

TASH makes a variety of joysticks which combine the standard four joystick movements with a fifth movement command input by either a pneumatic switch or push switches. These joysticks allow the user to move the cursor any direction and enter the information needed with minimal control. TASH's "Mini Joystick" is only 6" x 1.5" and weighs 10 oz.; the lever has to be pushed or pulled only 1/2" to cause cursor movement. ZYGO has a similar product, 4-Switch Joystick, which has a pushbutton switch as its enter device.

Still other users are able to harness their voluntary actions of grasping or flexing. For these users, there are elaborate glove devices and rubber cylindrical bellows which when "flexed" or "squeezed" signal the computer that they are ready to input information into the computer.

Finger Flex Switch is a product of Luminaud and consists of a switch built into a partial glove. Bending the fingers approximately 10-25 degrees activates the switch which will send the message to the computer. Luminaud also makes a gloved product called Magnetic Finger Switch with a magnet for those who cannot flex. The user moves a finger ever so slightly toward the magnet which sets the signal mechanism in motion. Products similar to Finger Flex (minus the glove) are Easy Action Hand Switch, a product of ComputAbility Corporation and Flex Switch by TASH. Both of these rubber-tipped bellows are attached to metal rods which rest in the user's hand and are activated when the user slightly flexes his hand.

Head Control

Prentke-Romich has a slogan for its HeadMaster switch—"If you can move your head...you can move your world." There is a segment of the severely disabled population which only has control of its head. For these people there are switching devices that when combined with others allow persons unable to use their hands to operate a computer. When operating a computer these disabled people are in control of information and therefore in control of their world. Several of the companies previously mentioned make head control switches.

FreeWheel System. Pointer Systems introduced the FreeWheel System in 1988 to allow a device without wires to move a cursor on a screen in front of the handicapped user (equivalent to a wireless remote control unit). A pointing device, controlled by a reflector connected to the eyeglasses and head-band of a user, moves the cursor by emitting infrared beams to a camera on top of the monitor.[7] The cursor will move on a keyboard-emulation display and allow the user to scan the display and enter the information he desires. This device is priced at just under $1,000.

HeadMaster. HeadMaster is a product of Prentke-Romich and takes the place of a mouse. The signaling device slips around the head (much like headphones from a radio) and measures the rotation of the head; it sends this measurement to the control unit, which in turn signals the cursor to move. Selection is made by either a sip or a puff or a push (depending on best controlled motion). This switching combination allows the individual the same access to the computer as a user of a standard keyboard.

Headband Switch and Head Switch. Headband Switch produced by ComputAbility and Head Switch produced by Luminaud Inc. work on the same principle. A headband, equipped with a switch that has a small paddle or lever, is placed around the individual's head. Luminaud requires that the paddle rest on the individual's head as wrinkling the brow will activate the switch. HeadSwitch's paddle must somehow be tapped to activate (turning the head slightly to hit against the special head rest).

The above list of switches is by no means complete as there is a switch that can be adapted to work with any voluntary movement the user can make (it is important that the device not cause him undue fatigue, compromise muscle tone or cause pain to vulnerable joints). As the user's needs change, the switching unit can be adapted as well so that he or she can use devices such as computers to his or her maximum ability.

As stated previously, switches are simply the translators for alternate forms of keyboard input. One still needs some type of "language" which the switch can acknowledge and translate to the standard keyboard language. The programs used by an individual are also subject to the ability of the user and finding the best application possible for that ability. Some of these applications involve: 1) direct scanning, in which a user "points to" the target items through a single action; 2) indirect scanning, in which the cursor moves from one character to the next, until a switch signals that the cursor is at the spot where the user wants input made; 3) Morse code, a method where the switches connect to an adapter that translates the dots and dashes into keyboard notations.[8] These packages are typically priced around $500, although the more sophisticated packages are priced higher.

Scanning Devices and Programs

ez-SCAN

ez-Scan is a product of Regenesis Development Corporation and can be part of a total access package called "Multi-Access Package." ez-Scan is software which allows any IBM-compatible program to be displayed in a split-screen mode, i.e., as the screen actually appears and as it is in the scanning mode controlled by ez-Scan. The scanning feature of ez-Scan will move the cursor as directed by the user using a switch and allows appropriate signals from these switches to be recognized as keyboard input features. ez-Scan will work with most single or dual switches, including sip and puff switches and modified joysticks.

ZYGO ScanWriter

The ScanWriter produced by ZYGO is a portable scanner which can be equipped to read (using a synthetic voice) aloud what is being scanned or allow the speech-impaired person to use the ScanWriter as his voice. ScanWriter allows the user to store commonly used phrases, words or letters in a special directory in the scanner. This could include a complicated "log-on process" for an online search service, thus enabling the person without dexterity to log-on without being "timed-out" by the system. ZYGO also has an interface for the ScanWriter which allows the ScanWriter to be used as a keyboard emulator.

ScanPAC with RealVoice

ScanPac is a portable battery-powered scanner, developed by Adaptive Communications Systems, which also acts as a communication aid in that the unit yields audio-output as it is scanning. It attaches to the front of the keyboard (but can also attach to a wheelchair mount) and can be accessed through most switching devices including Morse code and joystick. The user will activate the switch when the correct letter or combination is arrived at by the scanner. The unit comes with a software program that will allow the user to store and rearrange messages with 1 to 5 letters or numbers, which saves the user time and tedious movements as short commands (print, type, search) can be recalled and input with one movement rather than five.

Freeboard

Freeboard is a software program that can display an image of the keyboard on a separate display screen (which can be placed at a comfortable reading level). The program, developed by Pointer Systems, allows the software currently being used to continue to be displayed on the PC monitor while the user is able to activate his keys via a simple single switch, mouse, trackball, or head pointer by following the cursor on the display screen. If the user would prefer not to have the Freeboard screen on a separate screen, there are programs which allow the user to place the Freeboard's screen to the side of the program or above or below it. Should the user wish the Freeboard to disappear while reading a screen there are a "NEXT" and "BACK" command which allow him to do so. This software package is priced at just under $800.

HandiKEY Deluxe and Key Window

Prentke-Romich is the distributor of HandiKEY Deluxe and also of Key Window (they are designed by Microsystems Software). These are memory-resident programs that allow users of scanning switches to input information and make selections of computer programs. Key Window was designed to work with Microsoft Windows while HandiKEY was designed for use with DOS commands. HandiKEY has word prediction capabilities and speech output capabilities.

Morse Code

Satellite communications, computer codes and hi-tech devices have made Morse code virtually obsolete to most of the population. But for a group of computer users Morse code and its language of dots and dashes is the "hi-tech" method for alternate computer input. Users able to activate a single switch can "sip" and "puff" out a code and have it quickly translated to a keyboard language. There are several software packages available that will teach Morse code as well as the actual translators. These tutorials can and will be used by curious individuals interested in learning a special language.

Morse code learning software (priced under $100) is available from Personally Developed Software. There is a package called PC Morse Code which teaches Morse code basics as well as special symbols. The program allows the user to progress from a beginner's level of 5 words per minute to up to an advanced level of 60 words per minute (a sufficient data input rate for most entry-level clerical positions). The other package offered by Personally Developed Software is called PC Drills, and does exactly what its name implies—drills the user on each individual letter of the alphabet as well as abbreviations.

The Morse code interface programs are available with various features. All of these software programs will translate a simple switch activation to a key activation.

ezMORSE

ezMORSE, available from Regenesis Development Corporation, is bargain priced at $75 and will allow a single or dual "sip/ puff switch" user to create Morse code which the computer will accept as if the corresponding letter had been typed on the keyboard. The code set is based on the standard military Morse code set, with special mnemonic codes used for all other keys. Speed is adjustable by the user and there are pop-up menus that can be accessed if codes are forgotten. ezMORSE requires 64K of RAM as well as a port (any type can be adapted).

MorseK

Also bargain priced ($130), MorseK, a product of Kinetic Designs, is a highly versatile keyboard emulator that allows a user who accesses "mobile life" by switches (one to three) to interact with the computer by using Morse code. MorseK will work with all IBMs, including laptops, and offers a variety of options such as variable speed cursor movement, key repeat, super key mode and debounce delays. MorseK uses standard military code and is RAM resident. This program requires either a parallel or serial port for computer interface.

HandiCODE

HandiCODE is a product of Microsystems priced at $500 and falls in the mid-range of Morse code input devices. HandiCODE converts single-switch Morse code to standard keyboard keys; it will also translate the computer's non-alpha numeric keys and user-defined commands. A macro facility provides abbreviation expansion for frequently used keystrokes. The macro command ability of HandiCODE would allow a user to define log-on procedures thus saving the user from having to type repetitive input commands. HandiCODE comes with a tutoring program (PracticeCODE) and allows a user input range of 1-99 words per minute. HandiCODE can be used to control several speech synthesizers and can even input and access information in columns. There is also a deluxe version of HandiCODE available for an additional $200 that would give the user word prediction capabilities and abbreviation expansion.

Morse Code Plus—WSKE II

WSKE II, which stands for Words + Software Keyboard Emulator, is at the high end of the added features and price scale ($1,200). WSKE II is equipped with a highly intelligent word and letter predictor that provides the sip/puff switch user with dual word prediction, abbreviation expansion, automatic word endings, punctuation spacing and capitalization. This means that the user will not have any trouble inputting commands (there are some online systems for instance that have tricky log-ons that require the user to type the password or exit commands in capital letters which can be difficult with MORSE code) and sips/puffs can be saved for other tasks. WSKE will work with most speech synthesizers and has a "No Voice" option. This is one program that states that it will run transparently with all off-the shelf software programs including graphics programs.

Beyond Switches—LIAISON

LIAISON is a totally different type of computer interface, accessed by "pointer" switches. It is a product of DU-IT Control Systems. DU-IT's product yields the user "full capability" when using a computer workstation, which translates to user independence because he has the ability to use every function of the computer, the computer's peripherals and environmental control functions. LIAISON is itself a type of peripheral in that it is an individual unit (measuring 15" x 15" x 5", plus monitor) which stands next to the computer and translates switch inputs into computer functions. The LIAISON electronics box emulates the computer's normal input, and controls any other type of device that may be plugged into it. A keyboard of the user's choosing is displayed on the LIAISON screen as the user is working with his/her program on the PC screen; when choices need to be "typed" into the computer, the user "points" to the appropriate on-screen keys and LIAISON translates these to standard keyboard strokes. LIAISON does not use any of the computer's memory and allows the user to emulate keyboard, mouse or other graphical menu-driven programs, at the same time allowing the non-disabled a non-modified unit (see Figure 3). While priced at $3,500, the unit comes with an experienced staff of DU-IT technicians willing to spend time with prospective clients (or people who wish to understand computer switching access). This staff is committed to developing products that remove obstacles the disabled may encounter that keep them from achieving "relative independence...(inasmuch as) no one does very much without dependence on others."[9]

Touch Screens

Touch screens are quickly becoming part of the commercial world. We use them when we make a withdrawal from an automatic teller or make a purchase from some modern vending machines. They are used because they al-

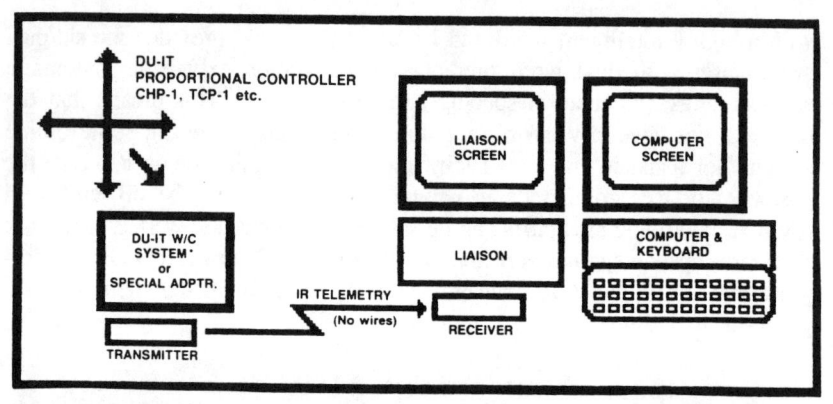

Figure 3. LIAISON is a unique device which makes use of an individual's abilities to allow him/her to access life.

low transactions to be represented by both words and illustrations, they prevent push buttons from sticking and they are user friendly. For the disabled user, however, they represent a feasible substitute to pressing keys. The touch screen can be laid on the PC's monitor or on a tablet (representing the monitor) positioned for easy access. Large highly sensitive target areas help the non-traditional keyboard user to work through menu-driven programs with greater ease. Several manufacturers of touch screen technology are willing to design touch screens at the user's request (each screen of a commercial software program requires a different overlay) and sell popular screen sets for programs such as WordPerfect. These products are reasonably priced (under $500 for complete sets) because they are designed by companies that also produce them for the commercial world.

TouchWINDOW

TouchWINDOW, priced at $300, is a product of Edmark Corporation. It is a simple plastic screen that fits over a monitor (with velcro), and is activated when the screen is lightly touched with a finger or stylus. Edmark has many "windows" available for word processing, spreadsheets and educational programs and will design customized programs. Edmark offers a TouchWINDOW language program for under $100 which allows users to create the applications needed by themselves. Many companies have created "touchwindows" for their products and a list of these is available from Edmark.

Touch System

Touch System, distributed by Carroll Touch Inc., is an overlay system which can make turnkey systems accessible to anyone capable of lightly touching a screen (which has highly sensitive sensors beneath it). The Touch System also works well with menu-driven applications which broadens its usage base, as log-on menus could be established or adapted for most software programs.

Touchware PC Translator

Newex's product, Touchware PC Translator, is a combination hardware and software product. The hardware is a mini-console incorporating a touch-sensitive LCD screen, which when touched instantly sends information to the PC. Sub-menus provide thousands of additional pre-programmed choices to work its way through intricate programs. Newex sells software to allow the user to develop his or her own menus.

UNMOUSE

UNMOUSE, by MicroTouch Systems, is a touch-sensitive tablet used for mouse emulation, graphic input and function key selection. The UnMouse is an absolute pointing device (i.e., the touch points map directly to corresponding points on the computer screen); touching the glass plate on top of the tablet (resolution of 1000 x 1000 touch points) moves the cursor to the desired location. Input is made by pressing downward on the tablet and by pressing a button to the left of the tablet (function key). MicroTouch Systems does not offer program customizing, but includes blank templates for the user for this purpose, as well as "how-to" instructions.

Touch screens allow the user who is able to "reach" and touch the easiest possible access to information. To fully utilize the touch screens, however, you should be ready to have one made for each application screen that the patron will use.

As stated in the opening of this chapter, the term limited mobility devices really means a "mixed bag" of technological devices used by people who need them to access life. These devices are the most intriguing and perhaps the most needed. While you may not be able to plan ahead in your purchases of them, be aware that they are available for a relatively small price.

Voice Input

Voice recognition is the newest form of alternate data entry and is not accepted by many of the rehabilitation professionals as being a legitimate form of data entry. But it is currently being used by some impaired users. This alternative input method takes a spoken command and translates it into keyboard commands. While this seems like an ideal method, problems faced by users of a voice recognition system are many. The voice recognition system must be trained to recognize the user's voice pattern for specific words and commands and once the computer learns the pattern, the user must always say the word precisely the same way with exactly the same intonations (not the easiest thing for a person with Cerebral Palsy to do). Most of the systems within financial reach of the population have a very limited vocabulary (500 words) which will help with the mechanics of programs (i.e., log-ons, menu selections). They cannot be taught words and subjects users wish to look up beforehand (i.e., a patron may need information on lithium for a special chemistry project—the word lithium would not be stored in a dictionary limited to 500 words). The systems with an unlimited vocabulary and tolerant to a person having a bad day and not enthusiastic in their speech are very expensive. Nevertheless, voice input is a viable alternate input method and one that can only get better and less expensive as it catches on in industry.

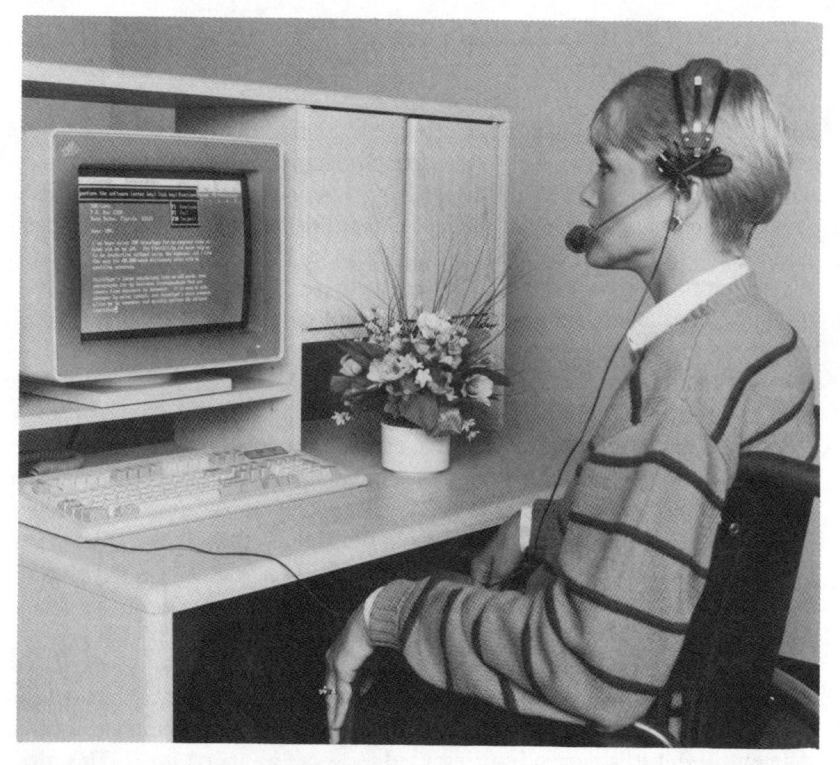

Figure 4. The DragonDictate has the appearance of a standard computer workstation, yet is much more intelligent.

DragonDictate

DragonDictate, priced at approximately $15,000, is the most elaborate and useful voice recognition system available as it turns any headset into a keyboard (see Figure 4). This product, which allows persons who cannot use traditional keyboards to verbally give commands to a PC, was not developed for the "physically disabled," but rather for the "time disabled" businessperson who did not have the time to dictate the material to a word processor and have an individual turn it into documents—DragonDictate was to do it all.[10] DragonDictate, a product of Dragon Systems, comes pretty close to doing this. DragonDictate was introduced in March 1990 and has the capabilities of recognizing 30,000 words for each user that it interfaces with, and can actually be taught that Miss M. says "to-may-toe" and Mr. N. says "to-mah-toe" when they both wish to type the word describing a zesty, red salad fruit. Additionally, DragonDictate will be able to learn speech pronunciation patterns and anticipate how the user will pronounce similar words, so that it will not have to be told that "po-tay-toe" and "po-tah-toe" are the ways in which Miss M. and Mr. N. will be pronouncing the reddish brown vegetable that tastes great baked or fried. DragonDictate allows the user to enter materials in windows or in columns. When the DragonDictate is equipped with a modem, the user can verbally command it to dial data banks without having to touch a key.[11] The device is expensive, but opens the information door to anyone who can speak within a few hours. Dr. William Salyers, Director of Easter Seals' Computer Assisted Technology Services, maintains that DragonDictate is actually better than a person at understanding and learning most speech patterns of even the most severely speech-impaired person.[12]

IBM PC Voice Activated Keyboard Utility

IBM is completely honest in its program description of the IBM PC Voice Activated Keyboard Utility when it says that it "allows control of unmodified, well-behaved application programs and provides voice recognition capability for commands and data input for these application programs."[13] IBM admits that all things must be normal for this utility to work and goes on to say that the user must be versed in DOS and programming aptitude as he is responsible for setting up commands, developing rules and remembering "grammar commands" within programs (dictates which commands are allowed at any given point).[14] This voice program is recommended only if you are planning a workstation for students to do homework with IBM application programs. Inquire to see if your dealer would be willing to include an IBM PC Voice Communication Option (part 6294771) and the PC Voice Activated Keyboard Utility (part 6280742) as part of a package deal.

IntroVoice III, V, VI

The IntroVoice products developed by Voice Connection Products are not nearly as sophisticated as DragonDictate but were developed to enable visually and physically disabled computer users to give basic operating commands to the computer. These recognition dictionaries are vastly smaller, the "ear" less sensitive and the price within the reach of the average user (price varies with size of dictionary recognition but all are under $750).

IntroVoice VI is a small 9 1/2" x 4" card which listens to the voice commands, translates and sends the equivalent keystroke data to the computer. The system then verifies the command by sending the command back to the synthesizer to be spoken. The IntroVoice VI is able to recognize 500 words/phrases and key the equivalent of 1,000 strokes. This allows a user to dictate a program log-on as well as work one's way through most of the program. While standard commands such as [type] CD\EE [return] [type] EE, [return] [down arrow] [return] will get users into the *Electronic Encyclopedia*, they will still need a way to tell the computer that they want information of St. Peter's Basilica. Both voice input and output can be easily integrated with any standard application program with no modification to the existing software, and once programmed by the user has an 98 percent accuracy rate.[15] The systems require a lot of memory: 60-64K for memory, 72-80K for recognition and 22K for text-to-speech synthesis. IntroVoice VI and other models (various prices/PC chassis models) are available from the manufacturer as well as the L S & S Group.

Voice Master Key

Voice Master Key is a product of Covox, a commercial voice synthesizer company. It is definitely designed for the budget minded (priced under $150) who needs voice access to the computer. Voice Master Key allows the user to store 16 macros in 16 fields, for a total of 256 macros. There is a total of 64 commands which can be assigned to activate a macro in any of the 16 fields, thus a single voice command can have several meanings, which works for and against the user (i.e., the user can store different macros in different fields which can be activated by the same word, which allows the user more working space within the memory field, but it also means the user has to be sure to define his field to get the correct action). The system is capable of learning its speaker's commands within an hour, displays the words it has learned around the border of the computer screen and verifies the speaker's input verbally. This program requires the installation of its software program and currently interfaces with a number of talking commercial software products including (with some manipulation) the *Compton's Multi-Media Encyclopedia*. Voice Master Key requires a spare slot in the PC for the plug-in circuit card and at least 64K of memory to run. Voice Master Key is available through Covox, LS & S and many mail-order computer suppliers.

Conclusion

There is a multitude of products and methods for inputting and retrieving computer information. Readers are urged to contact the vendors listed in Appendix 2 for more information about the products they intend to purchase and ask specific questions. Be prepared to tell the vendor the following:

1. Your intended patron group (i.e., students, seniors or senior students).
2. What you want to offer the intended group (i.e., information access via online, CD-ROM search only or the ability to do assignments as well).
3. The disabilities of the perceived audiences.
4. What equipment you have and would like to keep and the adaptive devices with which you would like to work.
5. If the workstation is to be shared between the "temporarily-abled" and the "disabled" computer user.
6. That you would prefer a demo of the product by an area representative (most have someone local) or have the right to return the item within 30 days if it does not interface as the manufacturer said it would.

Once you make your decisions on products to buy and have them installed, the next steps are easy and ones you are accustomed to for they involve providing the reference material and the encouragement to use the material provided. It cannot be stressed strongly enough that it will take more effort and a public relations campaign to convince disabled patrons that your library is open to them.

8

Technology to Assist the Deaf and Hearing Impaired

Most hearing impaired or speech impaired (i.e., inability to talk using their voice) library patrons do not require special adaptions to input information or extract information from printed material, which is still the material most used in conventional libraries. With the exception of a software program (SeeBeep) which alerts the hearing impaired computer user to auditory PC signals, the hearing-impaired user does not need any special adaptions to access computers or bookshelves. What both of these diverse groups do need, however, is an ability to communicate their needs to a world that is geared to react to verbal cues.

Most public libraries offer lectures, story hours, meeting-room use, videotapes and phone reference services not realizing that by acquiring a few pieces of hardware they would enable the hearing impaired user to access these services as well. Many public facilities also do not realize that by spending as little as $200 for a special phone, language impaired individuals can call the library with their questions.[1]

TDD Service

The easiest and most needed machine a library should purchase is a TDD phone. Basically a TDD is a keyboard that is used by a hearing impaired person, deaf user or a speech impaired individual to type a message to either an impaired or non-impaired user. The typed message goes through a phone line and appears in the viewing window of the other TDD. The hearing impaired user is signaled that the phone is ringing by a flashing light on the phone (many home users have remote signalling flashers as well so they do not have to watch a phone); non-impaired users prefer to interface the unit with an inexpensive phone to hear the ring. The TDD is extremely easy to set up; you simply plug the phone jack into the wall jack and it is ready to make and receive calls. Figure 1 is a typical setup of a TDD. Learning the usage of a TDD is equally as easy and can be self-taught although there is an excellent videotape "Using TTYs/TDDs" available from Sign Media, Inc. and Telecommunications for the Deaf, Inc. for $30.

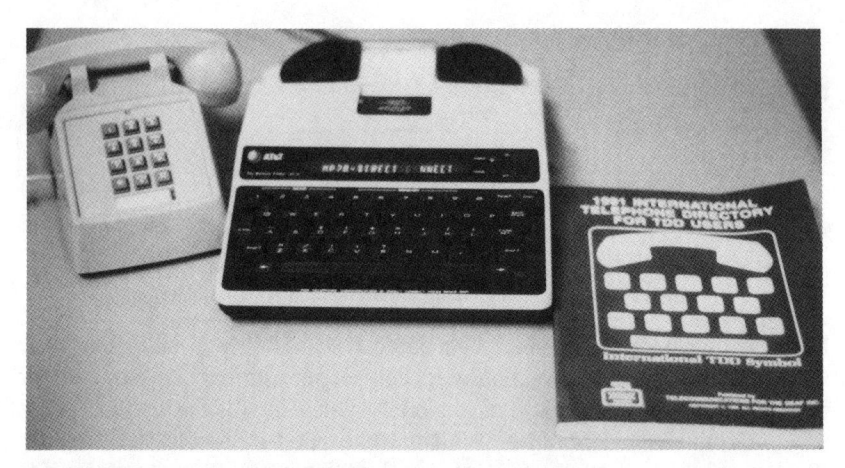

Figure 1. TDDs are as easy to install as a standard phone.

The system which uses state-of-the-art electronics (and can be used to make overseas calls as well as local ones) is fast and reliable. Proficient TDD users (the equivalent of good word processors), usually those skilled in American Sign Langauge (using abbreviations, and not skilled in syntactical rules of English), are able to send their sentences as quickly as a person speaking on a conventional phone. Typical abbreviations, which are logical and thus easy to learn, are shown in Figure 2.

```
TTY  - Teletypwriter (precursor to the TDD)
GA   - Go Ahead (I'm finished typing, your turn)
SK   - Stop Key, (Conversation over, hang up)
CUZ  - Becuase
HD   - Hold, Please
PLS  - Please
OIC  - Oh, I See
U    - You
UR   - Your
CD   - Could
Q    - Question Mark
R    - Are
NBR  - Number
SHD  - Should
TMW  - Tomorrow
```

Figure 2. Common abbreviations used for TDD communications

There is a rather sophisticated network in existence for TDD users as evidenced in the publication *"GA-SK Newsletter,"* a phone directory of TDD users and national conferences. These strong consumer statements encourage the industry to refine technology and keep prices low. There are several makes and models available, all under $500. The price differences are based on the display capability, reaction time of the key movements, buffer capacity and whether the unit has print and answering machine capabilities.

Krown Manufacturing

Krown Manufacturing was one of the very first companies to manufacture TDDs and is one of the industry leaders (AT&T uses this model with an AT&T logo). Krown presently makes six models with its own name: Portaview PV20 Jr., Portaview PV20D, Portaview PV20+, Memory Printer MP20, Memory Printer MP20D and Memory Printer MP40. The Portaview PV20 Jr. is the most basic of the TDDs; it does not come with a printer, but does have a printer port. The display is 20 characters in length. Portaview PV20D also has a 20-character readout but has a built-in printer that uses 2 1/4" thermal paper to record conversations, Portaview PV20+ has the same capabilities as the PV20D model, but has Auto Answer capabilities. The Memory Printer series has the same features as the Portaviews with the added capability of storing messages and phone numbers in the memory. The Memory Printer MP40 has all the previously mentioned features, plus a 40-character per-line printer. The units are priced from just under $200 to $600 (depending on features) and can be purchased from Krown, American Communications Corp., Harris Communications, Phone TTY and AT & T (whose service contract is with a Krown service center).

UltraTec Products

UltraTec produces eight models of TDDs that can be broken down to those that print and those that don't. The print models—Miniprint II, Superprint 200 and Superprint 400—are priced from approximately $375-$475. All of the units are portable and work with a battery pack or standard electrical socket. The Superprint 400 is the deluxe version of a TDD and has a built-in 24-character printer, 2,000 characters of memory, an auto-answering feature and direct connect keyboard dialing. The display window allows only 20 characters to be displayed at one time which makes the print feature desirable (it also saves you from having to take notes as the conversation progresses). The lower priced model, Miniprint II, is equivalent to your basic non-computerized phone, that is, it lacks the auto answer facility and stored phone directory.

The non-print models are priced from $200-$300 and are identical to the print models. These units are called the Minicom II, Minicom IV and the Supercom. If you need to save $200, these units will serve all your needs, but you will have to be able to take notes as you do with a normal phone call. UltraTec products are available directly from the manufacturer as well as Potomac Technology, American Communications Corp. and Harris Communications.

Additionally, UltraTec makes a large print display to aid the hearing impaired user who also has a visual impairment. The display unit offers the user a choice of lens colors to best suit his or her particular disability. The large-print display connects directly to the UltraTec Superprint 100-D TDD (a model that has special software to work with the large display) and enlarges all messages up to 10x. The display is so easy to read that even the non-visually impaired user can use it if s/he anticipates a long conversation.

Superprint TDD

Superprint TDD is a product of L S & S, and is an aid to the hearing impaired person who also has a visual impairment, or for the physically impaired user who cannot get close enough to the display window to read the message. The TDD attaches to a display unit which magnifies the messages 10x on a blue-green lens. The TDD itself is similar to those found in Krown's Portaview series and the UltraTec Minicom series and the package is identical to UltraTec's "Superprint" priced at under $650.

Higher-Tech Communications for the Hearing Impaired

UNI-PTC

If you cannot deal with the idea of acquiring one more piece of equipment and have a PC with a slot open, the UNI-PTC modem board and driver software is your answer. This item is priced at under $500, available from Integrated Microsystems Inc., and allows the user to communicate with TDDs and use the PC as he or she would use a telephone.

The jack that comes with the card plugs directly into the telephone jack and there is no need to have a conventional phone if the computer in which this is installed is monitored. When the phone rings the screen flashes on and off, signaling that someone is calling. If the unit cannot be monitored, then a phone will have to be connected to the PC to pick up the signal and read.

The UNI-PTC has the unique advantage of being able to store vast amounts of information that can be released by an impaired user with one keystroke. This feature would be really helpful to a physically impaired user who wishes to use electronic mail. This sophisticated device is available from Integrated Microcomputer Systems, Phone TTY and American Communications.

IBM PhoneCommunicator

The IBM PhoneCommunicator was designed by IBM's Special Needs Systems Group specifically to meet the needs of hearing and speech impaired persons. It will work with all IBM models and individuals can make or receive calls to/from deaf or hearing impaired users. Following PhoneCommunicator prompts, a hearing person uses a touch-tone dialing keypad to write a message to the deaf or speech impaired person. The user can then read what is written on the screen and type a response or use a prepared message, which is communicated through a synthesized voice to the caller (a big plus for the speech impaired user). The PhoneCommunicator also allows phone conversations to be printed and saved.[2] Priced at $600, this product is easy to use but has problems that must still be reconciled.

The PhoneCommunicator requires an analog telephone line to make and receive calls as well as a lot of memory. With 640K of memory installed in your PC, you are only able to run programs up to 256K; larger programs require the purchase of a memory management program, Software Carousel from SoftLogic. Another problem with PhoneCommunicator is that it requires a user wishing to transfer files to/from other system or to use it as terminal emulation to purchase an optional communications program, CrossTalk XVI, from Digital Communications Associates.[3] PhoneCommunicator is available through IBM Corp. and is supported by the Special Needs Center which developed it.

Electronic Phone Communications

While TDDs are sufficient for most users, professionals who have the need to use electronic mail need access to a network. Deafnet (Bell Communications Research) and DEAFTEK (GTEmail on Sprint) both have established networks that allow users to communicate with other networks such as USA, MCI Mail, Easylink, AT & T Mail and Internet. These networks are better accessed using a computer with modem and phone emulator because the message buffer is larger and file transfer is possible. They serve to translate messages left as speech to text for the hearing impaired person receiving and translate messages left as text to the non-hearing impaired.[4]

Closed Captioned Videos/Players

The fastest growing and most circulated audiovisual item is the video. Whether they are cartoons, classics or feature-length motion pictures, today's library patron demands them. This demand is also there among the deaf community as well. The technology for decoding television signals and videos is already present and used by a small segment of the deaf population (small only because of added costs and limited programming) and is called "captioning." The dialog/sounds are captured in American Sign Language or abbreviated text and shown to the deaf viewer through a "window" which can be seen only by someone using a decoder.

On October 15, 1990, President Bush signed into law the Televsion Decoder Circuitry Act of 1990 (PL 101-43) which mandates that by 1993 all television sets larger than 13" sold in the United States have a computer chip installed that will automatically receive and display captions of spoken words of various television shows, news programs, dramatic performances and movies. What this means is there will be more closed captioned programming on televison and as the hearing impaired world gets more accustomed to captioning the demand for closed captioned videos will also grow. Figure 3 illustrates the growth of captioning in a 10-year period.

There are many closed captioned videos being distributed now but the titles that are captioned are done at the whim of the motion picture companies. There is a lobby made up of screen stars such as Patrick Swayze, Ed Asner,

	1980-1	1989
COMMERCIAL (HR/WK)	16	130
CABLE (HR/MO)	4	680
SYNDICATION (HR/WK)	.5	86
COMMERCIALS	786	2829
HOME VIDEOCASSETTES	3	300+
SPORTS (HR/YR)	4	900+
LOCAL NEWS (MARKETS)	0	60

Figure 3. Captioning has seen real growth in all segments.

Glenn Close, Whoopi Goldberg and Meryl Streep who request that video viewers demand "closed-captioning" of all videos.

Libraries are urged to purchase videos and video playback equipment that can be enjoyed by all, especially if they are being used for programming. Decoders are available now from distributors such as Potomac Technology, Radio Shack (special needs catalog), J.C. Penney, Service Merchandise, Telecommunications for the Deaf, Inc. and American Communications Corp. The cost of a video recorder that will record closed captioned presentations as well as play back recorded ones is approximately $600 while the decoder for a television set is $200. Close captioned videos are the same price as a non-captioned video and a catalog of captioned videos can be obtatined from the National Captioning Institute.

Many libraries are now producing video tours of their library which can easily be captioned with software programs. Computer Prompting Corp. sells products that will do this simply called "Open and Closed Captioning Software" and "The Caption Maker." The first product allows the user to decide if the signed translation will be seen without a decoder (open) or with a decoder (closed) on a tape being produced. The latter product allows the overlaying of captions onto pre-recorded tapes (like over-dubbing). These items can be purchased from the American Captioning Institute, American Communications Corporation, Harris Communications and Phone TTY.

In-Person Communication

The hearing impaired community, (i.e., for the sake of this example, those who have some ability to hear amplified sounds) often have a hard time listening to programs because their disability prevents them from naturally screening out background noises to listen only to the speaker. The result is one big muttering. This situation can be easily alleviated for under $100 with the use of a device called Easy Listener.

Easy Listener

The Easy Listener system utilizes two components: the microphone transmitter which is worn by the speaker and the receiver which is worn by the listener. The microphone transmits the speaker's voice by an FM radio signal to the receiver worn by the listener (see Figure 4). The loudness of the speaker's voice is adjusted by a volume control similar to that on a transistor radio. The loudness and clarity of the speaker's voice will not be affected by distance, so the listener may sit anywhere s/he chooses. All the user has to do is: 1) put the headset on (if a hearing-aid wearer, the aid must be removed first), turn the unit on and wait for the speaker to begin; 2) when speaking begins adjust the volume control.

114 Library Technology for Visually and Physically Impaired Patrons

Identify the controls on the receiver.

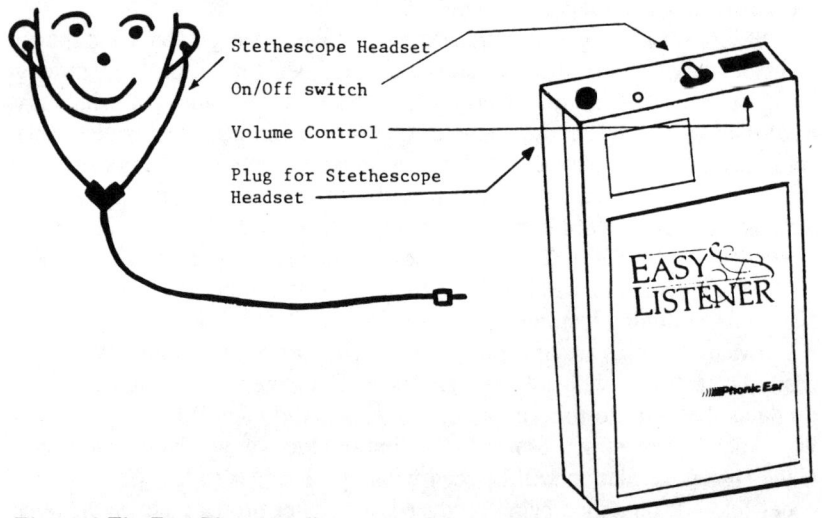

- Stethescope Headset
- On/Off switch
- Volume Control
- Plug for Stethescope Headset

Figure 4. The Easy Listener is lightweight and unobtrusive, yet yields clarity and understanding to the hearing impaired user.

Easy Listener is available from American Communications Corp., Harris Communications and Phone TTY. And, Radio Shack and Sears offer the same product in their Special Needs catalog.

Deafness is often perceived to be the "invisible handicap," one which goes unnoticed, much to the disadvantage of the person with the impairment. This group of individuals, however, can have access to most of your library for the price of a few pieces of equipment, costing under $1,000 total, and by remembering to purchase only captioned videos. These modifications do not require any expertise in equipment installations or computer use.

9

Putting Technology to Work in Your Library

Putting the system together was the hard part; deciding the format of the materials and collection development is the easy part. No doubt you already provide online database privileges to your non-impaired users as well as computer access to the library's catalog. It is a given (especially with A.D.A.'s [Americans with Disabilities Act] mandate) that you will also want to do the same for the impaired. In theory this is not a difficult task, but it does involve the purchase of a terminal equipped with a synthesizer and a staff willing to work to get the output.

Online Catalog Access

The Library of Michigan has made its online catalog to its collection of material (encompassing reference material, periodicals, newspapers, fiction with Michigan themes and genealogy) accessible by using an emulator board that communicates with the library's mainframe computer. This voice access system is called Answer Speaks and is composed of a Vert Plus voice synthesizer and Vista software which provides large-print access. Users are able to access the system independently after a few sessions.[1] Once the user finds the material s/he needs s/he either uses the Kurzweil reading machine or the Voyager Print Enlarger, also standard equipment in the Library of Michigan Catalog. Other libraries known to be using voice access to print library materials are The Special Needs Center of the Phoenix Public Library, The University of Texas in Austin, and the Cite des Sciences Mediatheque in Paris.[2] Many others are in the exploratory stages of this endeavor and are running into problems developing customized screens because of hardware conflicts between network interface cards and the speech cards. It is maintained, however, by the director of the Adaptive Technology Program of the Commonwealth of Massachusetts, that all these problems could be solved by the standard "trial and error method" of lifting and reinserting cards as dip switches are adjusted. This technique has successfully given speech to Banyan's VINES, Novell's NetWare and Articoft's Lantastic (admittedly after a flurry of flipping DIP switches and software gymnastics).[3]

CD-ROM Technology

The next thing you no doubt will do is give this group of people access to reference books and to do this all you have to do is acquire the most "disabled user-friendly" computer adaption to be developed since the personal computer itself—CD-ROM. David Holladay, editor of *Raised Dots Computing,* has said of the CD-ROM that: "For the sighted person, CD-ROM technology represents marginal improvements in search time, in cost, and in storage space. To a blind person, this technology represents volumes of text that can be read with a talking computer...previously we only dreamed about getting a massively indexed encyclopedia on a single disk and only dreamed about a service that would provide, on a monthly basis, full text of all general interest magazines."[4] Anita Richaume, a blind, doctoral student at the Universite de Lille III in Lille, France, pointed out several reasons why she believes CD-ROM is "the promise for the future" of learning for the blind and visually impaired because of the boolean search methods (i.e., even if works are transcribed on tape or braille, it is difficult to look for a word or sentence if needed) and the fact that the CDs are portable (e.g., even a dated collegiate braille or recorded dictionary cannot be be carried from residence to study location because of its size and the playback apparatus needed).[5]

The material from CD-ROMs has indeed made a difference in the type of service rendered to the users of the Cleveland Public Library's Library for the Blind and Physically Handicapped and various other libraries and rehabilitation centers. For example, patrons wanting information in braille on the Middle East are able to get current material, rather than being given material that is old and inaccurate; students needing a copy of the Periodic Table in large print to use for reference in a chemistry class are able to receive one in 16 pt. type.

Several special media libraries as well as individuals have been experimenting with this media with results that have been gratifying and enlightening. Each new title that is produced as a CD-ROM dramatically increases the amount of information available to special populations needing alternate access to information.

The basic steps to translate and use special media are straightforward. There will be variances for different CD-ROM titles and hardware as well as for the individual using the equipment.

Before being able to use any of them you will more than likely need to modify your autoexec.bat file and config.sys files. This is also easy but requires that a staff person logically think through the entire access procedure and answer questions such as: "Do I want to access the voice synthesizer by default (i.e., automatic activation upon log-on) or have it installed upon command?"; "Do I want to create menu access?" The following autoexec.bat file allows all programs to remain in residence and be summoned only when called upon. If a workstation is to be a shared one (i.e., used by disabled and non-disabled) then this is an example of the path you will want your boot-up to follow:

> AUTOEXEC.BAT
> line 1:   path=c:\dos;c:\bin;c:cdrom;c:\artic;c:\dots;c:\bkshlf
> line 2:   cls
> line 3:   \dos\mode com1:9600,n,8,1,p
> line 4:   \dos\mode 1prl=com1
> line 5:   Setcdpath=C:\bkshlf;F:\software;F:\book
> line 6:   Set CDRAM=
> line 7:   c:\mouse1\mouse
> line 8:   \bin\mscdex.exe /D:AMDEKCD /M:16

This file sets up the CD-ROM drive, an Artic Voice card, the Hotdots, the brailler, the Bookshelf, other CD-ROM software and a mouse.

CD-ROM programs are generally "memory greedy and file and buffer hungry" as are some of the adaptive software programs. The config.sys file listed below is an example of one which will allow the user of a PC with 1 MB of memory to successfully run a word processing program and the following CD-ROM titles: *Grolier's Encyclopedia, McGraw-Hill Encyclopedia of Science and Technology, WordCruncher, Microsoft Bookshelf, Search 450 CD-ROM (Eric Database and Schoolmatch), PDR, U.S. History on CD-ROM*, as well as software for the speech synthesizer and braille translator:

> line 1:   Lastdrive=Z
> line 2:   Buffers=20
> line 3:   Files=30 Device=C:\CDROM\AMDEK.SYS /N:1 /D:AMDEKCD
>   Device=ANSI.SYS

If you do run out of memory it is recommended that a memory manager be purchased to allow the screen reader to be stored into a higher memory.[6] "Quarterdeck Expanded Memory Manager," available through your local software vendor, works well with many speech-ware packages. Another alternative is to prepare a separate boot disk for each CD-ROM title rather than have all drivers stored on the hard disk drive.

If the workstation is to be used solely by the impaired user, menus could be set up to directly take the user to the CD-ROM programs, conversion programs, etc., which makes access easier. The autoexec.bat file and config.sys files illustrated below are used by the Special Needs Center in Phoenix to run a menu system:

AUTOEXEC.BAT
Line 1:   path=C:\dos;c:\sonix:c:\vocalize;c:\wp;C:\batch
Line 2:   c:\CDROM\MSCDEX.EXE /D:AMDEKCD /M:8
Line 3:   set CDPATH=C:\BKSHLF; D:\Software; D:\Book
Line 4:   cd\
Line 5:   set CDRAM=
Line 6:   cd\sonix
Line 7:   sonix /I=7
Line 8:   tts
Line 9:   cd\
Line 10: cd\vocalize
Line 11: artic/!c4
Line 12: /!k4/!f5
Line 13: /f1init.set:
Line 14: cd\
Line 15: auto
*

Config.sys
Line 1:   Lastdrive=G
Line 2:   Files=20
Line 3:   Buffers=20
Line 4:   Device=C:\CDROM\AMDEK.SYS /N:1 /D:AMDEKCD

Whichever method you choose to set up your CD-ROM access point, once in the search, retrieval and translation will be easy and straightforward.

Large-Print CD-ROM

The large-print application simply involves loading the large-print program (stored on your hard drive) and then loading the CD-ROM title. The

```
                    Special Needs Center
    Select Item      1. Load WordPerfect
    Move Arrow       2. Load Electronic Encyclopedia
    Page UP/Down     3. Braille Conversion & File Transfer
    More Help        4. Load WordPerfect Without Voice
                     5. Load MicroSoft Bookshelf
                     6. Copy a Disk, A: to A:
                     7. Load Grab Brag Menu
                     8. Exit
```

Figure 1. This menu is representative of the series of four menus used by patrons of the Phoenix Special Needs Library, Phoenix, Arizona.

search can then be made and information accessed and printed if needed. The print should be a clean bold type devoid of "serifs," and at least 14 pt. type. The following photographs illustrate the process a visually impaired user would use to execute a search (note: the products listed are used because of author's familiarity).

Load Large-Print Program (ZoomText). ZoomText is memory resident, so the user only has to type the command: ZoomText. Instantaneously the letters appear at the default magnification of 2X (see Figure 2). The user

```
TYPE:      C> ZOOMTEXT

           and

           ZOOMTEXT
    TEXT MAGNIFICATION SOFTWARE
 COPYRIGHT (C) 1987-90 BY A1 SQUARED:
           VERSION 3.23
```

Figure 2. The command to retrieve the software program is typed in and the program appears instantly.

chooses the attributes including the magnification to a size that is easier to read, from the default setting (see Figure 3). At this time the user can also make changes such as type of display magnification (i.e., entire screen showing magnified text or left/right side, top/bottom of screen magnified while normal print is displayed) and scanning process.

```
ZOOMTEXT HAS BEEN LOADED INTO MEMORY.
PRESS [ALT] [INS] KEYS TO POP-UP MENUS.

C>              ZOOMTEXT

                ZOOM
                MAGNIFY
                WINDOW
                REVIEW
                FONT
                EXIT
```

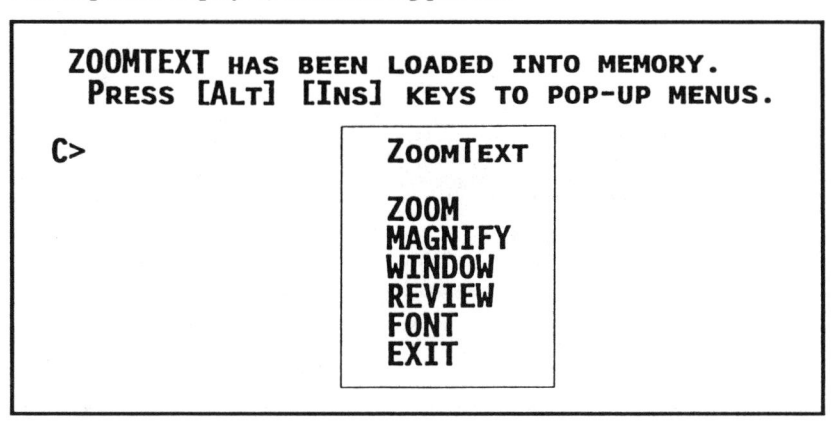

Figure 3. The menu system allows the user to adjust attributes to suit his or her reading needs.

120   Library Technology for Visually and Physically Impaired Patrons

The user now simply loads the CD-ROM title and does the needed search (see Figure 4).

```
ZOOMTEXT HAS BEEN LOADED INTO MEMORY.

PRESS [ALT] [INS] KEYS TO POP-UP MENUS


C>CD\CONCISE

C>CONCISE
```

Figure 4. After the software has been loaded, the patron proceeds with loading the CD-ROM title and doing his search.

When the user finds the material he wants he can decide to print or read it. If he is experiencing problems using the attributes he originally chose, changes are easily made (see Figure 5).

If the user decides to print the text, s/he would choose the font on the printer and make any other possible page format changes within the CD-ROM program to generate the proper page layout for the larger text. It may be necessary to choose a horizontal format as in Figure 6. The font cartridge manual will tell the display pitch for the print chosen.

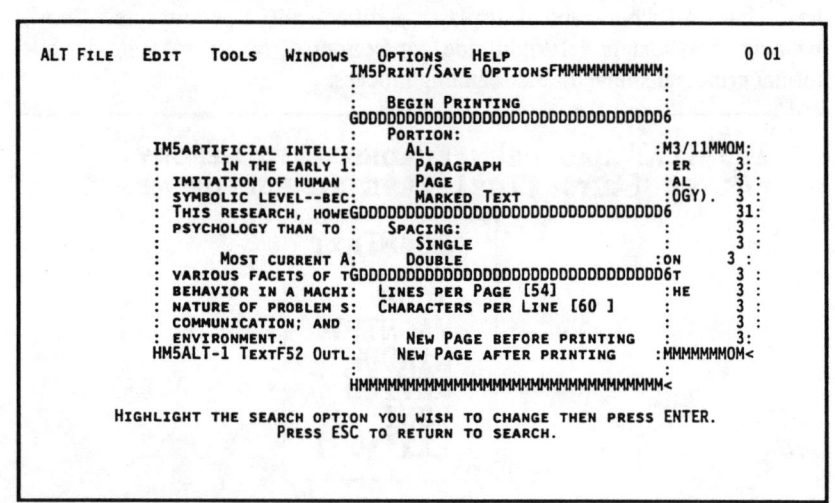

```
ALT FILE   EDIT   TOOLS   WINDOWS   OPTIONS   HELP                        0 01
                                    IM5PRINT/SAVE OPTIONSFMMMMMMMMMM;
                                    :   BEGIN PRINTING                :
                                    GDDDDDDDDDDDDDDDDDDDDDDDDDDDDDDD6
                                    :   PORTION:                      :
                  IM5ARTIFICIAL INTELLI:   ALL                    :M3/11MMOM;
                  :     IN THE EARLY 1:   PARAGRAPH              :ER     3:
                  : IMITATION OF HUMAN :   PAGE                   :AL     3 :
                  : SYMBOLIC LEVEL--BEC:   MARKED TEXT            :OGY).  3 :
                  : THIS RESEARCH, HOWEGDDDDDDDDDDDDDDDDDDDDDDDDDDDDDDD6  31:
                  : PSYCHOLOGY THAN TO :   SPACING:                    :  3 :
                  :                    :   SINGLE                      :  3 :
                  :    MOST CURRENT A: :   DOUBLE                   :ON    3 :
                  : VARIOUS FACETS OF TGDDDDDDDDDDDDDDDDDDDDDDDDDDDDDDD6T   3 :
                  : BEHAVIOR IN A MACHI:   LINES PER PAGE [54]        :HE   3 :
                  : NATURE OF PROBLEM S:   CHARACTERS PER LINE [60 ]  :     3 :
                  : COMMUNICATION; AND :                              :     3 :
                  :   ENVIRONMENT.     :   NEW PAGE BEFORE PRINTING   :     3:
                  HM5ALT-1 TEXTF52 OUTL:   NEW PAGE AFTER PRINTING    :MMMMMMMOM<

                                    HMMMMMMMMMMMMMMMMMMMMMMMMMMMMMMMM<

         HIGHLIGHT THE SEARCH OPTION YOU WISH TO CHANGE THEN PRESS ENTER.
                      PRESS ESC TO RETURN TO SEARCH.
```

Figure 5. Some titles allow you to adjust the lines and spacing within the program, others must be made with the printer control.

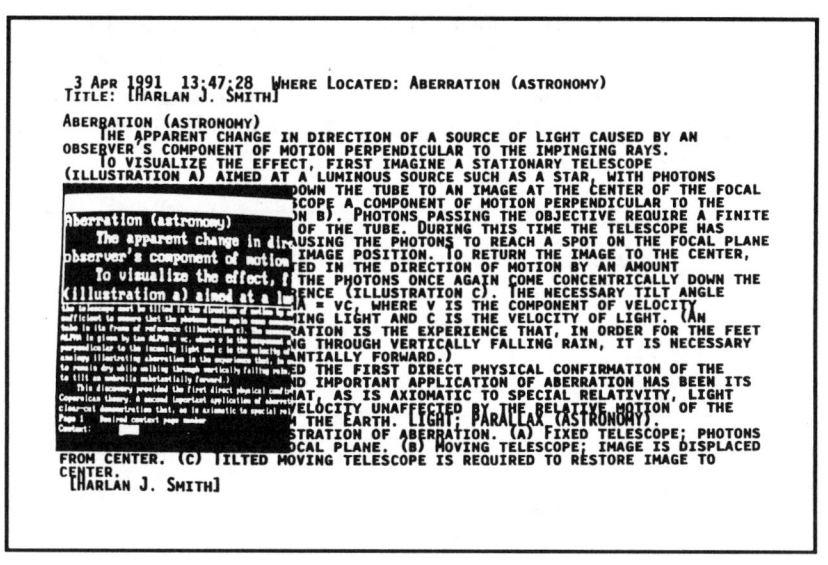

Figure 6. Remember that horizontal printing is acceptable.

Most CD-ROM programs do not allow for manipulations within the program to change the lines per page and characters per line; choosing a horizontal font is the easiest solution to capturing the complete text in print.

Printers and CD-ROM programs develop situations that require the user to issue commands to the printer to produce readable and complete text. *WordCruncher*, for example, advises users to edit the printer command string for their program if using a laser printer. The user need not know DOS to do this but must have patience to accurately type the string given.

Voice Access from CD-ROM

Speech output is easily accessed by the impaired by following two basic steps: loading the speech translator and loading the CD-ROM title. Loading the speech translator is a matter of recalling it via DOS command and as soon as the translator is loaded, the user will immediately receive an auditory cue for each key pressed and for everything that is visually seen on the screen. Although this sounds ideal for someone who cannot see, adjustments must be made to tell the screen reader that you do not want to hear, for example, the function cues read on every screen or that the area of information you wish to read begins at the grid intersection of 40 and 40 and ends at 40 and 80. The user is also able to change the pitch of the voice (or in the case of some synthesizers the actual voice itself), and the rate of speech read (see

Chapter 5). The following steps illustrate a typical search process for voice access:

First, the user would load the speech synthesizer simply executed by recalling the software from hard disk drive; the user would then make any adjustments (see Figure 7).

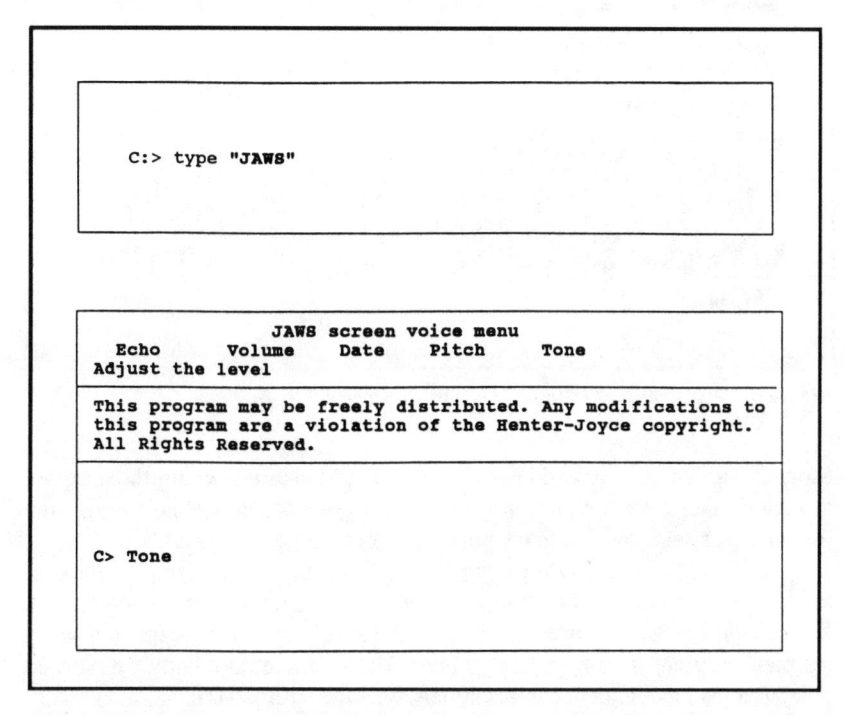

```
C:> type "JAWS"
```

```
              JAWS screen voice menu
   Echo       Volume     Date     Pitch      Tone
Adjust the level
```
This program may be freely distributed. Any modifications to this program are a violation of the Henter-Joyce copyright. All Rights Reserved.

```
C> Tone
```

Figure 7. Speech access can be as simple as turning on the computer and selecting items off the menus.

After the user makes the changes which allow him to listen to the synthesized speech in a manner pleasing to him, he is ready to listen to the screen text.

If the user is not familiar with adjusting windows, all information he wants read may be saved to hard disk. This is done by using the save function of the CD-ROM program and retrieving it after following the basic load step of the synthesizer program. The "TYPE" command is used to retrieve and read the entire file which was saved: C> "TYPE" NAME OF FILE

Virtually all CD-ROM titles can be accessed with voice output using this method, as long as a few things are kept in mind. First, the more graphical the interface, the less translatable it is to speech. A screen full of icons, pictures and overlapping windows becomes gibberish to screen-reading programs seeking clean ASCII.[7] Figure 8 illustrates items that will cause a screen reader to have difficulties in reading. These screen notations are items that commonly appear on screen displays, but they are not recognized by screen readers as standard English-language notations and as a result will cause some screen readers to abort reading as the reader becomes confused.

1. ********** OR -----------
   REPEATING SYMBOLS

2. TEXT WHOSE FORMAT   IS
                        COLUMNS
                        RATHER THAN
                        BEING PRINTED
                        ACROSS THE
                        ENTIRE SCREEN

3. TEXT IN WINDOWS RATHER THAN USING FULL WIDTH OF SCREEN

4. BRIGHT, HIGHLIGHTED BAR MENUS WHICH FLASH AS CURSOR MOVES THROUGH OPTIONS

5. TEXT WITH ILLUSTRATIONS

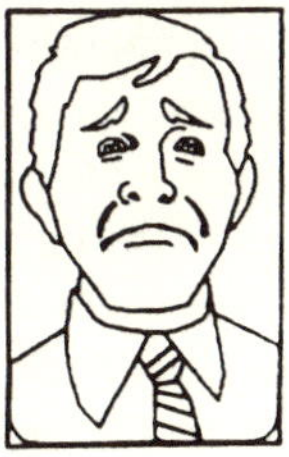

Figure 8. Items that may cause trouble in translation to special media

Braille Access to CD-ROM

Direct braille access to all CD-ROM titles is possible using a paperless braille display unit or indirect access can be had by printing the information in braille. Both procedures are accomplished in a straightforward manner. Judith Dixon, Ph.D., Consumer Relations Officer for the National Library Service, is the owner of over 20 different CD-ROM titles and uses the paperless braille approach to access CD-ROM titles. She has not had any problems with the titles she has purchased and suggests adjusting the required color VDT to as "black and white" as you can get it to allow the braille translators to function at their best. With the unit in Figure 9, braille access is made easy as the CD-ROM title is loaded and the user is able to read the information without any manipulation.

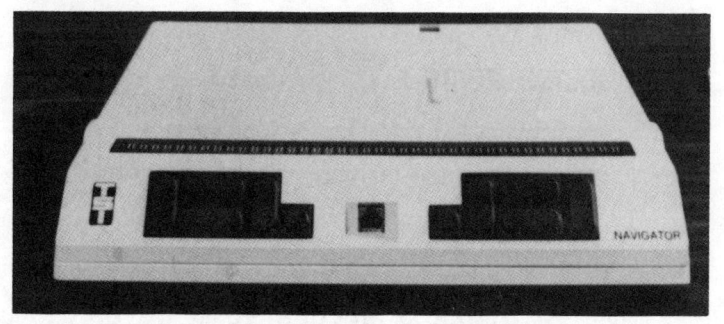

Figure 9. The paperless braille display unit, Navigator, slips under the standard keyboard amd allows the blind computer user access to all messages and information appearing on the computer screen. Photo courtesy of TeleSensory Products (TSI).

Braille Search and Print

The braille search and print procedure assumes that the user is searching the CD-ROM database by voice or large-print access or that the search is being conducted for the individual by a sighted person. The information found is always saved onto the hard disk and must be taken through a translating program (see Figure 10).

The translating software is loaded and when it is installed the commands are given to translate and format (see Figure 11). The document is printed using either the translator commands or the DOS command to print.

Virtually All Titles Will Translate

In Appendix 3 you will find a listing of CD-ROM titles that a small group of CD-ROM alternate input and output users have successfully used.[8] These titles offer the librarian as the disabled's "information seeker" to get current material. While CD-ROMs offer the most up-to-date and economical

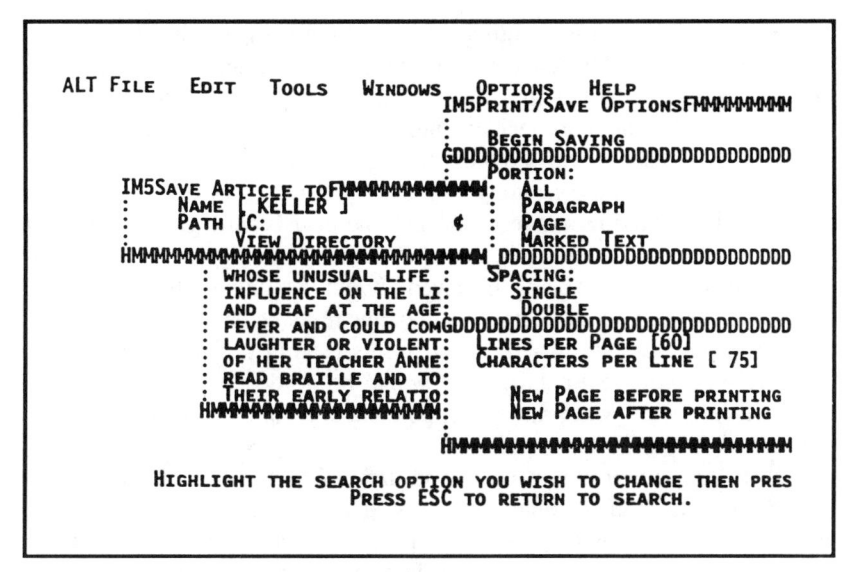

```
ALT FILE    EDIT    TOOLS    WINDOWS  OPTIONS  HELP
                                      IM5PRINT/SAVE OPTIONSFMMMMMMMM
                                      :  BEGIN SAVING
                                      GDDDDDDDDDDDDDDDDDDDDDDDDDDDDD
                                      :  PORTION:
IM5SAVE ARTICLE TOFMMMMMMMMMMMM;  ALL
    : NAME [ KELLER ]            :  PARAGRAPH
    : PATH [C:           ¢       :  PAGE
    :  VIEW DIRECTORY             :  MARKED TEXT
HMMMMMMMMMMMMMMMMMMMMMMMMMM DDDDDDDDDDDDDDDDDDDDDDDDD
    : WHOSE UNUSUAL LIFE  :  SPACING:
    : INFLUENCE ON THE LI:    SINGLE
    : AND DEAF AT THE AGE:    DOUBLE
    : FEVER AND COULD COMGDDDDDDDDDDDDDDDDDDDDDDDDDDDDD
    : LAUGHTER OR VIOLENT:  LINES PER PAGE [60]
    : OF HER TEACHER ANNE:  CHARACTERS PER LINE [ 75]
    : READ BRAILLE AND TO:
    : THEIR EARLY RELATIO:     NEW PAGE BEFORE PRINTING
HMMMMMMMMMMMMMMMMMMMMM:         NEW PAGE AFTER PRINTING
                                      :
                                      HMMMMMMMMMMMMMMMMMMMMMMMMMMMMMM
        HIGHLIGHT THE SEARCH OPTION YOU WISH TO CHANGE THEN PRES
                       PRESS ESC TO RETURN TO SEARCH.
```

Figure 10. To translate CD-ROM information to braille simply save the information to the hard drive.

form of reference information for the "computer literate" (or those willing to become literate) disabled, one should not forget using information that may be available on diskette or online searching possibilities.

There are some excellent self-instruction diskettes available for the learning impaired and the hearing impaired. These two groups do not face

```
PLEASE ENTER ONE OF THE FOLLOWING OPTIONS:

1) IMPORT FILE FROM WORD PROCESSOR
2) TRANSLATE PRINT INTO BRAILLE
3) FORMAT FILE PRIOR TO OUTPUT
4) OUTPUT TO EMBOSSER OR PRINTER
5) GLOBAL SEARCH AND REPLACE
6) BACK TRANSLATE BRAILLE INTO INKPRINT
7) QUIT

ENTER A NUMBER>:DOTS 2 3 4, LPT1

CHOOSE OPTIONS TO TRANSLATE, FORMAT,
AND PRINT BRAILLE OUTPUT
```

Figure 11. Choose options to translate, format, and print braille output.

any physical obstacles to inputting and retrieving computer information; the exception being that the deaf cannot hear the signaling audio sounds made by some programs and DOS itself. This problem has a simple solution called "SeeBeep." This memory-resident utility, priced at $20, is a product of MicroSystems and provides on-screen messages each time the PC sounds an audio beep. Both the learning and hearing impaired benefit greatly from the repetitious tutoring nature of the PC; the deaf benefit greatly from language drills and the learning disabled are able to learn more effectively if information is read as it is being displayed. If your institution offers a hands-on, free-access or staff access fee-access to online research databases, then equipping the search terminal with disabled access is a must. If it is a library staff member doing the research, all that would be needed is braille translating software or a large-print printer (it is possible to record the synthesized reading, although the results are poor).

Another option is membership in national bulletin boards and LANS. Using specially adapted computers, the visually and physically impaired can solicit aid in problems they may be experiencing and help others. There are bulletin boards of this nature established in all areas of the country. Case Western Reserve University in Cleveland, Ohio, maintains numerous bulletin boards through its Information Gateway and one is specifically geared toward adaptive devices (announcements of new products) and clues to solving adaptive computer problems. It is not uncommon to see personnel from NASA's Lewis Research Center assisting a Health Sciences bulletin board (disabled users group) user or a Health Sciences member using alternate access answering a question from someone in the NASA engineering department.

A highly regarded LAN was started by a blind rehabilitation engineer, Donald Breda, in Boston and uses an Opus BBS system dedicated to the use of speech and other special needs. Like Gateway, it is common to see sighted and non-sighted sharing information and working to solve problems. The listing in Appendix 4 is a sampling of networks formed to specifically serve as a forum for users of alternate access technology and those assisting these users to discuss information on products (success and failures). Remember that any database bulletin board accessed by a computer is one that is accessible to the disabled.

The Ideal Library—Your Library—Hardware

The ideal accessible library would include a fully accessible PC capable of allowing a visually or physically impaired user access via:

1. Audio input and output with synthesizers.
2. Large print input and output using software and special fonts (large print keytops would be evident).

3. Braille input and output using paperless braille displays, braille translators and printers (braille locator dots or the complete alphabet on one keyboard).
4. Large and small alternate membrane keyboard access; software programs that would reconfigure multiple keying functions; programs to accent input via Morse code or sip/puff, toggle, push, scan, point switches.

The PC workstation would also be connected to an optical scanning device capable of reading any print material and relaying the information to the user in a format which he or she could access independently.

In this "ideal" accessible library, one would also find a closed circuit television camera for use by those patrons simply wanting to read their newspaper or determine the amount of their heating bill.

This "ideal" accessible library would also be fully staffed to assist anyone needing training on any of the equipment to receive it for as long as it takes them to feel comfortable using it.

This "ideal" accessible library is possible only if money is no object, as it would cost at least $30,000. Since most libraries have frugal budgets, most will only be able to build their accessible library a unit at a time. Quite a few libraries have made much progress in using technology to make themselves more accessible and the following libraries surfaced as leaders at an American Libraries Association workshop held in summer 1990.[9]

Boston Public Library has developed an ACCESS Center that provides large-print and talking books, closed captioned videotapes, players and computers with voice and braille access. It provides the patrons with a braille embosser as well.

Seattle Public Library has a program called LEAP (Library Equal Access Project), which includes a full-time project coordinator and the following equipment: Kurzweil Reading Machine, video print enlarger, and a VersaBrailler plus PCs with large-print and synthetic speech access. They recently purchased a CD-ROM player for the PCs. The Seattle Public Library has also installed TDDs on many of the public service desks, purchased many closed captioned decoders and videotapes and an FM loop system for participation of deaf patrons in public meetings. Seattle relies on volunteers to make LEAP work.

The Skokie Public Library, always a notable leader in the area of accessibility, serves persons with disabilities through the Skokie Accessible Library Services (SALS). The library does not require the user to be a resident of Skokie and provides all who enter with services such as an IBM PC-XT that can be accessed with large print, voice or braille. The library also has closed circuit television print enlargers and closed captioned video players which it loans for home use. A Kurzweil Personal Reader is part of its equipment inventory and the library relies on volunteers to train users to become proficient in the use of the technology. Additionally, the building has a meeting room with sound amplification for hearing impaired audiences.

The Special Needs Center at the Phoenix Public Library is also an acknowledged leader in providing technology to aid the print disabled patron. In addition to having an extensive collection of print and video material on disabilities and assistive devices, it has a Kurzweil Reading Machine and adequate staff to train new users. A paperless braille display unit and a braille embosser interface with an IBM PC to give the user access to CD-ROM material and the Arizona Public Library's online print catalog.

The Florida Regional Library for the Blind and Physically Handicapped is using technology to bring braille into all libraries in the state. The library has a dedicated group of volunteers who transcribe print books into braille using the same computer technology that has been described in this book. The information is stored on diskettes, which can be shipped to participating libraries and circulated to a patron who has access to a printer or a refreshable braille reader. This project is in its final evaluation phases, working out the bugs that tend to surface with such a far-reaching project.

Perhaps the most far-reaching model of library service to the disabled was developed by the Chancellor's Office of the California Community Colleges along with the State Department of Rehabilitation, Health and Welfare, and other agencies. They collaborated to operate a High Tech Center Program for people with disabilities. The High Tech Centers are presently located at 51 community colleges, three state universities, one University of California campus (Northridge, which actually developed the foot-mouse) and three high school Regional Occupational Programs. They are equipped with state-of-the-art technologies that allow 150 trained professionals to assist 5,000 students in acquiring information and knowledge.[10]

Other academics on the cutting edge of technology for the disabled include the University of Nebraska-Lincoln which maintains a center for disabled students and is presently creating a LAN by which students can access CD-ROM databases and use OCR devices; the University of Missouri-Columbia maintains a 100-station general access computer lab which trains disabled students (and students who wish to work with the disabled) and service providers in the allied health industry and has as one of its goals "equal access to information"; and the University of North Texas which through multi-departmental cooperation has Kurzweil readers, braille printers and speech synthesizers as part of the Department of Computer Science.[11]

These examples serve only as ideas for a direction to take. Any type of effort you make is a statement of developing a positive outlook. The effort you make this year may be as simple as installing a TDD phone, but the small group of users who will use it will be appreciative of the fact that they were able to receive the same phone reference service as the non-hearing impaired. The effort you make may be similar to that of the Warwick Public Library (RI) which purchased a VTEK-Voyager, CCTV. It reported that it found the equipment to be of great help to visually impaired users wishing to use reference materials.[12] The step you take may be similar to those of Chester County Library (PA) System and the Ridgewood Public Library (NJ), both of which were recipients of a Lions Club donation of a Kurzweil Personal Reader. The director of the Chester County Library, Jean Heibeck, said that her library received inquiries about the Kurzweil Personal Reader before it was installed and have been training patrons in its use on a regular basis and for a variety of reasons.

An Easier Route—Ready-Made Systems

For those of you who do not feel comfortable putting a computer system together but have the funds, there are several workstations that come packaged and ready to offer immediate access to visually and some physically disabled users. While you will still have to add items such as a CD-ROM player or a membrane keyboard or a scanner (depending on the package), the basic interfaces are already made. These stations are available from Henter-Joyce, LS & S and Talking Computer Systems and may be available from several of the larger companies that sell a diverse selection of computer equipment rather than specialized items such as synthesizers or enlargers.

Ultimate Reader I

The Ultimate Reader I is available from L S & S. It comes complete with a PC/AT compatible computer, monochrome monitor, two floppy drives and a hard drive, serial and parallel ports, the latest MS-DOS, a scanner (Ultimate Reader), Recognition Card, HP Scan Jet, WordPerfect 5.1, WP Sift Software and PC Braille (braille translators), Artic Visions Software and Synthesizer and a braille embosser. By purchasing this unit (priced at $15,000) your patron will be able to scan printed documents and convert them to synthesized speech or braille, plus be able to use a word processing system and read any material available on disk. If you wish to offer reference service beyond this you will still have to purchase a CD-ROM unit (this is actually the easiest of the interfaces) and if offering online searching, a modem. If you wish to offer a refreshable braille display you would have to purchase the unit separately.

Access PC Color Systems

L S & S also offers packages for the large-print user, speech synthesis user and the braille user. All of the units are priced at approximately $4,500 and include an AT computer and the appropriate software and hardware to render the format requested. For instance, the Speech Computer System comes installed with an Artic Speech card, a monitor, DOS, a letter-quality daisy wheel printer and an applications software package; the braille system package has a braille software translator and the daisy-wheel printer comes with a platen capable of pressing out braille dots (since dots are not crisp, this format of brailling will be minimally legible to most braille readers). L S & S also has an option plan that lets you purchase additional options for $600 each when one complete package is purchased.

Excellence Reading System

Excellence Reading System is a package of quality products. The features include a "loaded" IBM compatible (1 Mb of RAM, a 40 Mb hard disk drive, a 101 Keytronics keyboard, a 5 1/4" 1.2Mb and a 3 1/2" 1.44 Mb floppy disk drive, one parallel and two serial ports), a monochrome video monitor, and an installed JAWS speech system, Prose 4000 Text-to-Speech synthesizer, the Arkenstone scanner and HP document feeder. The system comes configured for JAWS and WordPerfect 51. The system is priced at $11,000 and is available from L S & S. It will allow the user access to print documentation and any material available in disk format. To use CD-ROM technology, online searching or to render any service in braille or large print, additional equipment and software would have to be purchased separately. This system has room for growth of CD-ROM titles as it has a large amount of memory.

HeadStart III-CD

Henter-Joyce has an answer for the CD-ROM buyer, as it sells PCs with CD-ROM players (complete with an extensive software package of 17 useful titles, most of which are public domain, but include *Grolier's*, *Microsoft-Bookshelf*, and *Microsoft-Stat Pack)*. The package, called HeadStart III-CD, includes a PC which is IBM compatible and comparable to that which comes with the Excellence Reading System. The package is priced at approximately $3,000 and can have an Accent PC synthesizer installed for approximately $750 extra. Braille and large-print devices would have to be added for those who use those formats. Henter-Joyce offers a 48-hour service contract and provides on-site consultant service at a per-day rate of $400 plus expenses.

Talking Encylopedia

Talking Computer Systems offers a package deal that combines an Artic synthesizer and a CD-ROM unit with one title for a little over $1,500. This company also sells large-print and braille interfaces and would be able to put the proper package together that would give you voice, large print and braille access to all CD-ROM packages. You would still need to secure keyboard access for the physically handicapped from another source. Talking Computer Systems has the expertise of Joe Lazzaro, a frequent user who has written many articles on the subject of computer access.

Collection Growth

All of the aforementioned package deals make it easy to get started. Continuing is indeed a cautious but rewarding task. Jack Moore, president of Open Access Publishing, suggests that you ask the following questions when purchasing software for adapted systems.[13]

1. Does the publisher/distributor have a software preview policy which enables you to "try before you buy?" There are some programs which may be affected by the unusual interface.
2. Does the publisher offer technical support for the product? While the publisher may not even begin to understand what you are doing with alternate input/output methods, if a problem does arise it would be helpful to know if it's the software or the hardware.
3. Is the program one that you would also buy for the non-disabled? With the exception of educational drills for certain disabilities, material should be on the same intellectual level providing stimulus and growth.
4. Is the documentation clearly written and organized so that instructions can be rewritten in another format? The information should be straightforward to facilitate someone rewriting the instructions in another media (i.e., braille large-print).
5. Does the program contain too many graphics? As mentioned previously screens that are pleasing to the eye are not necessarily pleasing to interfaces.

6. Can the program be operated with a limited number of keys? If it can't, will the program work with an Adaptive Firmware Card of PC AID?

If possible it is advisable to avoid using a software program to emulate multiple key functions simply because it is one less loop to travel. Be sure to try all functions with your adaptive devices when you purchase them. He also implied that unless you are an expert, you will no doubt make some mistakes. Rest assured that the old adage "You learn from your mistakes" applies to adaptive technology as well.

Mr. Moore's statements on software are also true for hardware purchases—unless you are an expert you will make some mistakes. Most of these mistakes can be easily corrected by some type of "patch" job at a low cost. The companies mentioned in this book, while profit-making ventures, are in it not only for profit but because they want to make a difference in impaired persons' lives. It cannot be stressed strongly enough to ask them your questions and not to rely on your local computer hardware vendor unless your contact there is willing to do background work and contact adaptive technology manufacturers to learn what type of interface this special equipment requires (i.e., if interfacing a PC with an OCR scanner, what is the port requirement, how much RAM is required, is there a slot open for recognition card?). After your questions are answered, join the ranks of those who offer "knowledge for all."

Staff Training

Even though the disabled live in all communities and, in theory, are mainstreamed in the educational community (i.e., public schools) with the end purpose being societal assimilation, we have not seen mainstreaming carried forth into our workplace, our social organizations, or into our libraries. As a consequence of this unintentional segregation (reinforced with stereotyped characters in books and film), misconceptions and misgivings about the disabled are formed and maintained.

Staff Sensitivity Training

These feelings often stem from a lack of information or understanding about a particular disability and a desire not to offend the person with the disability. Unfortunately, in the desire not to offend this very thing happens, even in the intellectual environment of libraries. Your staff will no doubt be in need of a sensitivity training session with the goal of making them realize that the disabled do not necessarily "require special services, but they may need special, creative ways of accessing the same resources provided to everyone."[14]

Several methods are currently being used by libraries. One method involves having a workshop in which videotapes are shown followed by small break-out sessions led by persons who are actually disabled. Another method is to show videotapes and provide the staff with bibliographies of books about various disabilities.

The first method is the preferred method (suggested readings can still be distributed) because it serves to take away the element of the "unknown" and makes the staff aware that the disabled patron is not someone to be feared, that the disability is not contagious and that, while they may make a "faux pas" when they are rendering service, the mistake will be treated the same by the disabled person as it would be by the non-disabled (i.e., some will respond belligerently and some will be understanding). It is not difficult to find good, disabled public speakers to come to your workshops, as many organizations, such as the National Federation of the Blind, have a public speakers bureau with sensitive people willing to share experiences in a stimulating and non-threatening manner and emphasize ideas brought out in videos.

Good choices of videotapes include "People First," produced by Library Video Network, Baltimore County Public Library and distributed by the American Library Association, and "A Place Where I Belong," produced by the Greater Vancouver Public Library Foundation and distributed by the Services for Handicapped Persons division of the National Library of Canada.

"People First" is 38 minutes long and comes with a discussion guide that encourages the staff to think and better understand the barriers, physical and attitudinal, that the disabled face when they use libraries. Rather than scolding the viewer, the video offers positive suggestions and solutions to situations which may occur when disabled persons visit the library.

"A Place Where I Belong" is a 16-minute display of positive interaction between disabled children and public librarians. In addition to showing hearing and visually impaired children interacting with the library, it also shows a child using a wheelchair, entering a public library, and using DecTalk to introduce herself to the librarian. The librarian makes her welcome, as she would any child, and allows her to feel that she does indeed belong in the public library even though she cannot talk or walk without technological assistance. The video is open-captioned thus the viewer is also given a brief introduction to sign-language.

If you cannot have disabled commentators speak at your training session, be sure to make an effort to include a readable packet of information for each staff member. Many professional organizations have free or inexpensive materials available which do not require that the individual spend a lot of time reading but do give enough information to make the reader feel more secure and correct when addressing and serving a disabled patron. The Ohio Library Association has recently published a set of seven pamphlets covering library service to various disabilities and older adults. These pamphlets were developed on a high school comprehension level to encourage all staff to read them. The American Foundation for the Blind also has easy-to-read pamphlets on such topics as "What do you do when you meet a deaf-blind person?" Please see the bibliography for other reading and video suggestions.

Develop Guidelines for Service

It is suggested that guidelines for services to individuals with disabilities be formulated to assure that staff knows what is expected of them. Some organizations have specific guidelines of service as part of their operating manual.[15]

Guidelines will be unique to your organization. They may include specifics on how to introduce the technological equipment in your library to the patron, how to answer the TDD, and basics such as when to offer your services. Staff will appreciate knowing what is expected of them and the patrons will appreciate knowing what they can expect from the staff and the library. Never make unreasonable demands of the staff as this may lead to resentment which will carry over into the delivery of services.

In addition to contacting organizations that have guidelines, there are several books that can help you and your staff develop guidelines that you will feel comfortable with, notably *Meeting the Needs of People With Disabilities* (Velleman), *Library Manager's Guide to Hiring and Serving Disabled Persons* (Wright), and *Person to Person: Community Awareness of Disability* (Gething).

General Guidelines

There are some general guidelines that should always be followed when serving the impaired library user, but remember, impaired people are individuals with varying degrees of independence; approaches which work with one individual may not work with another. The guidelines listed below are very general, and are of the "courtesy" type.

1. Offer assistance as you would to anyone entering your library. You may directly ask if the person needs help with their wheelchair or may ask the blind person if they would like an orientation tour to the library. Note: It is perfectly acceptable to ask questions "What would you like to see (or look at) today?" of a visually impaired patron or give direc-

tions such as "Walk down to the end of this row, which is about 5 feet long, and turn left and it will be 2 feet to the right" to a person using a wheelchair, as visually and physically impaired persons frequently use these terms themselves. When giving directions to the blind person, always include a measurable reference.
2. Noticing a disability is perfectly acceptable, deciding what the person with the disability needs is not. Always ask the person what type of assistance he or she needs, but do not ask personal questions.
3. If the disabled patron who wishes assistance is accompanied by an "able-bodied" person, talk directly to the person requesting assistance.
4. If the person is hearing impaired it is perfectly acceptable to ask the person if they lip-read. If they do lip-read, be sure to move into a well-lit area and position yourself to directly face the person who is watching. Avoid placing hands or any other objects around your mouth and give explicit examples when dictating individual letters. For instance, always say "B" as in boy, because Bs are often heard as Ps. If the hearing impaired person does not lip-read or is having trouble lip reading, do not hesitate to communicate with the person by writing out your conversation or using your video display terminal, equipped with a word processor or a TDD, to carry on a conversation by keying in the words.
5. Be aware of hidden disabilities. A person with a cane or guide dog is obviously blind, but persons with impaired vision may not even be wearing glasses but will bring reading material closer to their eyes on a regular basis. A person who is hearing impaired (rather than deaf) may be able to hear if the person is speaking directly facing him but will not be able to hear someone approach from behind. A person who is learning disabled will be able to drive himself to the library and hold intellectual discussions of the highest caliber, but may not be able to read and copy a call number from the computer.
6. If you know that a disabled person is in the library, alert other staff members where they are on case an emergency arises. Be direct when doing this. Do not use gestures as the disabled person will sense you are speaking about him or her and wonder exactly what is being said.

7. Staff should always be patient, but not condescending. Like any patron, once the disabled person is oriented to the equipment and feels relatively comfortable using it, s/he should be left alone, with the advice of "ask the assistant on duty if further help is required" (specific instructions on the person's location should be given).

Training the Patron

As the staff becomes comfortable following the general guidelines of service to disabled library patrons they will be comfortable with introducing and instructing the patrons in the use of the high-tech equipment you purchased.

Training will require one-on-one sessions. For instance, if in an academic setting you will not be able to train all your incoming impaired freshmen at the same time using an overhead projector, someone will actually need to orient each one.

Before training can begin, however, the staff must be comfortable with the use of the equipment. They should know how the equipment works, they should know who could make use of the equipment, and when to encourage the patron to try it. When they are ready to train the user, the following basic guidelines will be of help:

1. Instructions for using the equipment should be transcribed in an alternate medium for quick reference by the user. For instance, it would be helpful to have the instructions for the CCTV done in large print and posted in an accessible location near the workstation and braille intructions and product descriptions in a notebook by the computer station. Additionally, items such as CD-ROMs or diskettes should also be labeled in large print and braille.
2. When giving instructions to the impaired user keep in mind that he or she will be assimilating information with one (or more) fewer senses; help him or her work with the senses they do have. The visually impaired person should be told specifically that "the switch to turn on the monitor is the top dial on the right side of the screen."
3. Do not set unreasonable time limits for learning how to use the equipment. If training time is limited because of limited staff, try to solicit volunteers to help with the persons needing extra help. These volunteers may come from the group of users you have already trained (most will be glad to share their expertise).

These guidelines are meant only to serve as a starting point from which you and your staff will grow. One hard and fast rule to offer, though, is "never be afraid of failure." Although adaptive technology may seem intimidating in the beginning, once learned, it will be the most rewarding lesson ever learned. All the various pieces will fall into place and make sense (as well as work). Training individuals to use the high-tech devices will become as second-nature as training staff to work the "ready-reference desk" or students to use the public access catalog. Maybe easier.

10

Future Growth of Adaptive Technology

Most of us will agree that this is an exciting time to be living in. The advances that technology has wrought in the last 10 years have been truly amazing. Although not designed with the disabled in mind, computers, for instance have become tools for many. There are even greater inventions on the horizon that promise more for the disabled than presented in this work. An occupational therapist at Ranchos Los Amigos Medical Center said, "We look at technology needs from an interdisciplinary approach. If someone can move any body part, if it is only an eyebrow, we can use adaptive programming for computer access. If a standard piece of equipment does not exist, we can create it...the individual introduced to a computer...reacts as if given a key to independence."[1]

On the horizon are products such as Dexter, a robot hand which will aid people who are both deaf and blind. The hand, still in a testing stage, will interface with a computer and translate ASCII typed into the computer to finger-spelling which the hand will actually spell out in the palm of the deaf/blind person.[2]

Another product, Eyegaze, allows even the most severely impaired to communicate and "live."[3] Eyegaze (see Figure 1) was designed by LC Technologies for the small handful of people who cannot voluntarily control any muscle consistently enough to communicate at all. This device allows the user who can control his or her eyes to not only operate a computer, but also to control his or her entire environment. Eyegaze would never be purchased for the public sector (priced at $30,000, it comes complete with a voice and training by two nurse-technicians), but is offered in this discussion to reiterate the fact that knowledge can and should be open to all people able to think and reason. The Veterans Hospital conducted tests on quadriplegic veterans and Joseph Binard, national director of the VA's prosthetic and sensory aids services, said, "I am always looking for new technology to help the handicapped over their disability...it seems to give the severely disadvantaged the chance to regain the use of computers...and (life)."[4]

Also developed but not yet marketed is a braille mouse (Model II) which, when connected to a PC, allows the braille users to read text stored in

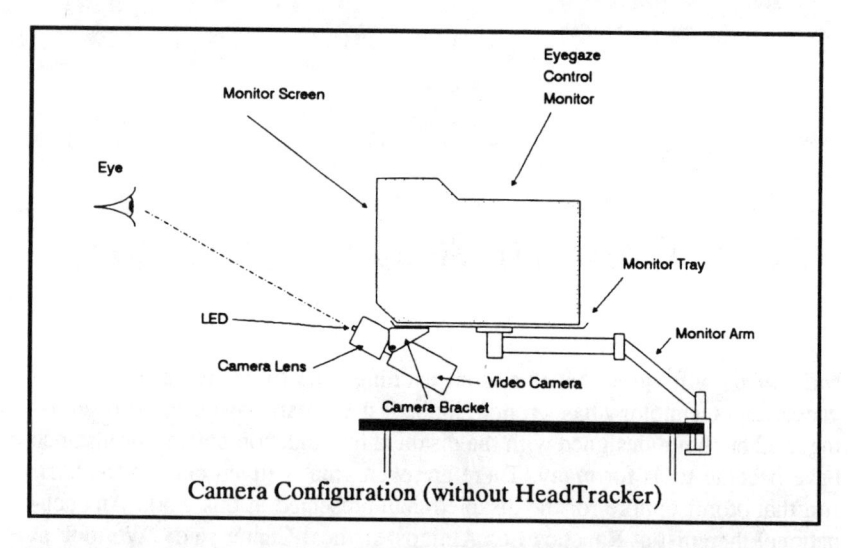

```
                    Eyegaze
                    Control
   Monitor Screen   Monitor
          \          /
   Eye     \        /
    ◁- - - - -[ Monitor ]
                   |      \
                   |       Monitor Tray
         LED       |      /
           \       |     / Monitor Arm
   Camera Lens -[ ] /  /
                 [Video Camera]
          Camera Bracket
   ━━━━━━━━━━━━━━━━━━━━━━━━━━━━━
   Camera Configuration (without HeadTracker)
```

Figure 1. Based on aerospace technology, Eyegaze allows the person who can focus only his or her eyes to access technology and control his or her environment. Source: "Eyegaze Computer System for the Physically Handicapped," LC Technologies, Inc., 1989.

electronic memories. The braille mouse was developed at NASA's Langley Research Center by H. Douglas Garner and should retail for approximately $200. The mouse is moved along a flat surface from left to right, the cursor on the screen travels from character to character and converts each electronic character it sees to the braille equivalent. Pins raise and lower in the mouse signalling the braille reader what is being read. This is refreshable braille in a most economical (both dollars and space used) format.[5]

Elliot M. Schreir, director of the National Technology Center of the American Foundation for the Blind, recently made predictions on existing technology.[6] He asserts that: "Technology will be improved and finicky OCR scanners will read handwriting, newspapers, poor quality print and will incorporate high-contrast, color-flat panel displays for the magnification of images. These scanners will also eventually be able to interpret symbols and graphic displays." Schreir further projects that "improvements in synthetic speech will be made as this technology becomes mainstreamed into life" and that as it gets more sophisticated it will also "help the functionally illiterate communicate in the print world."

ADA Mandates the Future

We will see more companies willing to make minor modifications to their products to accommodate the disabled, as the Americans with Disabilities

Act (ADA or Public Law 101-336, 42 USC 12101-12212) begins to be phased in. There will no doubt be an increase among those who are impaired demanding equal access to employment and information and the impaired will legally be able to challenge individuals and institutions that do not grant them this equality.

The "Findings and Purposes" section of the ADA declared that discrimination against individuals with disabilities is "a serious and pervasive social problem which persists in such critical areas as employment, public accommodations, education...communication, recreation and access to public services...which results in discrimination, including outright intentional exclusion, and consequently segregation and relegation to lesser service, program, activities, benefits, jobs, or other opportunities."[7]

While a discussion of ADA is not the purpose of this document, the readers should be reminded that the contents of this book are what the ADA is all about. Title I of ADA mandates that, unless there is "undue" hardship it is indeed "unlawful to discriminate against individuals with a disability in regard to job applications procedures, hiring and advancement and the privileges of employment."[8] Software screen enlargers would enable a visually impaired word processor to become competitive for a secretarial position; a paperless braille display or speech synthesizer interfaced with a PC would enable a blind individual to compete for a job at a "quick" reference desk using encyclopedias found on CD-ROM or perhaps at a business information desk where phone number inquiries are often the main query.

Title II mandates that "no individual with a disability shall, by reason of such disability, be excluded in or denied the benefits of the services, programs, or activities of a public entity (herein defined as any organization which meets the essential eligibility requirements for receipt of services provided by a public entity, i.e., public funds), or be subjected to discrimination."[9] To comply with this mandate, a library should have closed-captioned videos, if it has a video collection; a library should offer a telecommunications device for the deaf, if it offers phone reference service; if a library has a print reference collection, it should be accessible by the visually impaired either by CCTV or an optical scanner or an attempt should be made to at least offer some reference service on CD-ROM with braille, large print or synthesized voice adaptions; if a library has an online catalog that is for public use, then all the public should be able to use it, which means it should be wheelchair height, have a membrane keyboard and have an alternate output option (this would not necessarily mean all stations would have to be equipped in this manner).

Title III of the ADA addresses architectural discrimination against individuals by private entities, and extends itself to include nongovernment-funded schools (both elementary, secondary, college), and any "museum, li-

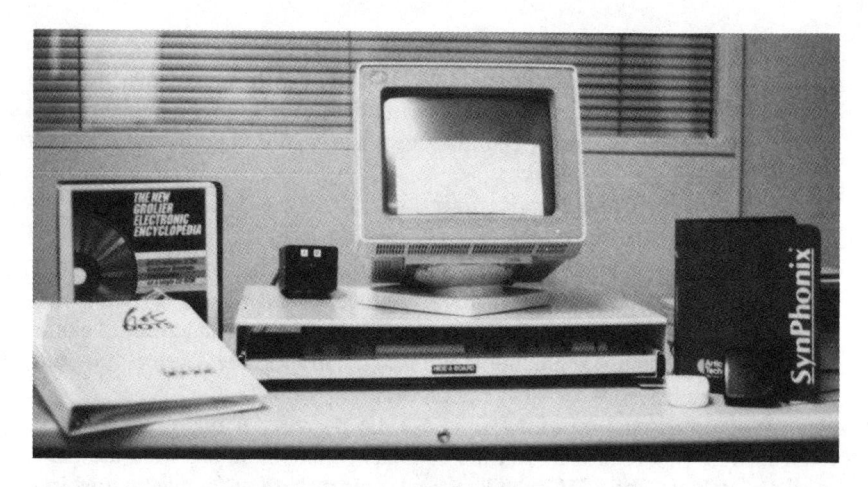

Figure 2. Technology gives everyone equal access to information.

brary, gallery, or other place on public display or collection." It states that "no individual shall be discriminated against on the basis of disability in the full and equal enjoyment of the goods, services, privileges, advantages, or accommodations...and that all of these be afforded to an individual with a disability in the most integrated setting appropriate to the needs of the individual."[10] For libraries, this should mean allowing everyone to physically enter the building if they desire; heavy doors may need replacement, ramps may have to be added, elevator panels should have braille notations—in other words extend all technology, be it computer technology or architectural technology, to include all people.

An adaptive technology technician was quite candid with me when she said, "You know I find libraries the most inaccessible public institutions in existence, which really upsets me because I tend to think of libraries and librarians as fountains of knowledge and it hurts to think that they have the opportunity to let me in and don't...maybe I'm just guilty of stereotyping librarians as being better (smarter) than the average person, which is equivalent to the general population viewing the disabled as being less smart than an ablebodied person." Is she right or wrong with her assessment of libraries? That is a question each library and librarian will have to answer on an individual basis. Making ordinary tasks "do-able" for the disabled requires money and effort, but it is possible. It requires you to find the money. Appendix 5 offers some possible sources of money so that you and your staff can make a commitment to carry this out. This may call for the personnel department to conduct sensitivity training for the staff; for the public relations department to constantly let the disabled public know that the library is now one which they can use; and for the staff to be willing to learn new technology and train new users.

All the effort expended will be worth it; you will be reaching out to a most eager user group. Anita Ross, vice president of IBM Canada, summed up the promise of technology when she said, "For most of us technology makes things easier, but for people with disabilities it makes things possible."[11] Her statement was echoed by Al Gayzagian, blind since birth and presently working as director of corporate reporting (using a synthesizer) for John Hancock Insurance, when he said, "With a PC, I have access to a great deal of data that I never had...before it was a great deal more awkward to get information, and there was some that I simply didn't have access to."

Let your library be a fertile place where all can learn and grow together. Let it ascribe to the doctrine of equal access to information.

Appendix 1:
Registered Readers (Thousands) of the NLS Network

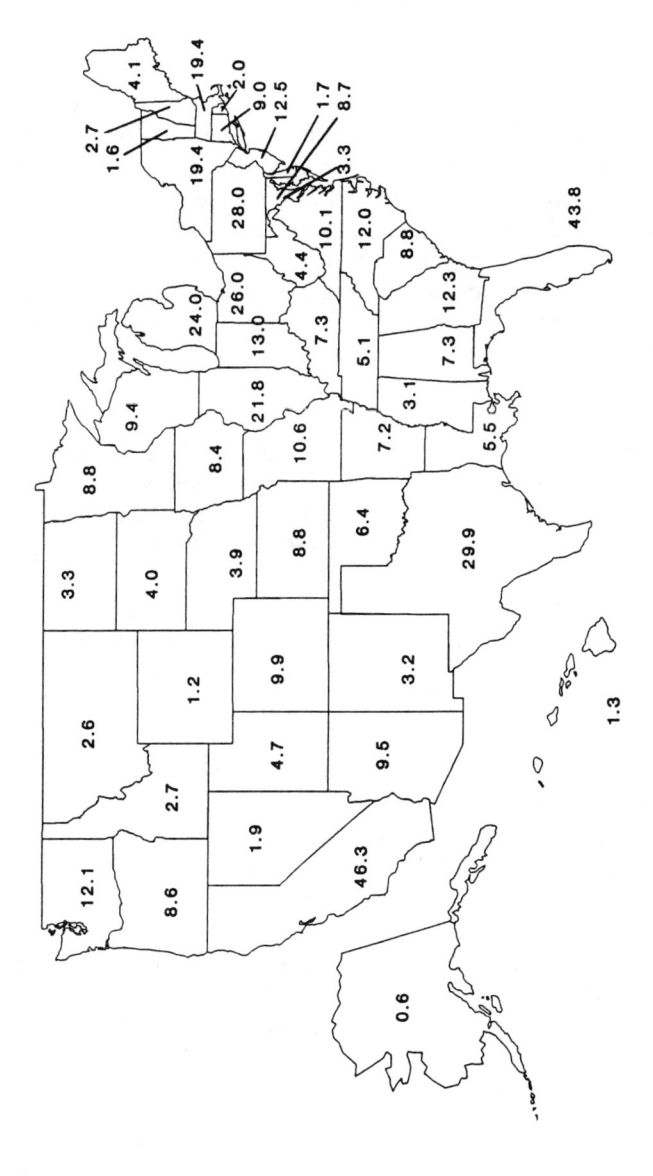

Appendix 2:
Vendors and Distributors of Technological Devices for the Blind and Physically Handicapped

Note: This listing is by no means complete nor is it an endorsement of these particular organizations. Interested purchasers are encouraged to consult IBM's National Support System's *Resource Guides* for a more thorough listing. Other sources of information on vendors include: *Computer Technology for Handicapped Persons-Some Questions and Answers* (National Library Service), *Sources of Products for Blind and Visually Impaired Persons* (American Foundation for the Blind) and *Closing the Gap Resource Directory: A Guide to the Selection of Microcomputer Technology for Special Educatiog* (Closing the Gap).

A-1 Squared
1463 Hearst Dr., NE
Atlanta, GA 30319
(404) 233-7065

Ability Systems Corporation
1422 Arnold Ave.
Roslyn, PA 19001
(215) 657-4338

Ablenet
1081 10th Ave. SE
Minneapolis, MN 55414
(612) 379-0956 or (800) 322-0956

Adaptive Communication Systems
354 Hookstown Grade Rd.
Clinton, PA 15126
(412) 264-2284

Adhoc Reading Systems
28 Brunswick Woods Dr.
E. Brunswick, NJ 08816
(800) 783-3210

AICOM Corporation
2375 Zanker Rd., Suite 205
San Jose, CA 95131
(408) 922-0855

ALA Video
American Library Association
50 E. Huron St.
Chicago, IL 60611
(800) 545-2433, press 8

American Captioning Institute
5203 Leesburg Pike
Falls Church, VA 22041
(703) 998-2400

American Communications Corp.
1040 Roberts St.
East Hartford, CT 06108
(203) 289-3491

American Printing House for the Blind
P.O. Box 6085
Dept. 0086
Louisville, KY 40206
(502) 895-2405

American Thermoform, Inc.
2311 Travers Ave.
City of Commerce, CA 90040
(213) 723-9021

Ann Morris Enterprises, Incorporated
46 Horseshoe Lane
Levittown, NY 11756
(516) 796-4938

Arkenstone, Inc.
540 Weddel Dr.
Suite 1
Sunnyvale, CA 94089
(408) 752-2200 or (800) 444-4443

Artic Technologies
55 Park St., Suite 2
Troy, MI 48083-2753
(313) 588-7370

ARTS Computer Products, Inc.
145 Tremont St., Suite 407
Boston, MA 02111
(617) 482-8248

ATR Computer Tec.
P.O. Box 58
Wierton, WV 26062
(800) 359-5923

AT&T Special Needs Center
2001 U.S. Rt. 46
Suite 310
Parsippany, NJ 07054
(800) 233-1221

Bell Communications Research
435 South St.
Morristown, NJ 07960
(201) 829-2000

BIT (Boston Information Technologies)
52 Roland St.
Boston, MA 02129
(800) 333-2481

Blazie Engineering
3660 Mill Green Rd.
Street, MD 21154
(301) 879-4944

Bloorview Children's Hospital
25 Buchan Ct., Resource Centre
Willowdale, ONT.
M2J459 Canada
(416) 494-2222

BOSSERT Specialties
P.O. Box 15441
Phoeniz, AZ 85060
(800) 776-5885

Calera Recognition Systems
2500 Augustine Dr.
Santa Clara, CA 96054
(408) 986-8006

Carroll Center for the Blind
770 Center St.
Newton, MA 02158
(617) 969-6200

Carroll Touch, Inc.
P.O. Box 1309
Round Rock, TX 78680
(512) 244-3500

Celexx Corp.
2535 Seminole
Detroit, MI 48214
(313) 925-9368
  or
3404B Redcoach Trail
Lexington, KY 40502
(606) 272-3210

Centigram Communication Corp.
4415 Fortran Court
San Jose, CA 95134

CLEO, Inc.
3957 Mayfield Rd.
Cleveland Heights, OH 44121
(216) 382-9700

ComputAbility Corp.
40000 Grand River Rd.
Suite 109
Novi, MI 48050
(313) 477-6720

Computer Prompting Corporation
3408 Wisconsin Avenue
Washington, DC 20016
(202) 966-0980
(202) 966-0886 (TDD)

COPH-2
2020 Irving Park Rd.
Chicago, IL 60618
(312) 866-8195

Covox, Inc.
675 Conger St.
Eugene, OR 97402
(503) 342-1271

Crestwood Co.
P.O. Box 0406
Milwaukee, WI 53204-0606
(414) 461-9876

Data Cal Corp.
531 E. Elliot Rd.
Suite 145
Chandler, AZ 85225
(800) 233-0123

Designing Aids for Disabled Adults (DADA)
249 Concord Ave. #2
Toronto, ONT.
M6H 2P4 Canada
(416) 530-0038

Digital Equipment Corp.
146 Main St.
Maynard, MA 01754-2561
(800) 832-6277 or (603) 884-8990 (NH)

Don Johnston Developmental Equipment
900 Winnetka Terr.
Lake Zurich, IL 60047
(312) 438-3476

Dotson Enterprises
1901 N. Bayland St.
Pensacola, FL 32501
(904) 432-0894

Dragon Systems
90 Bridge St.
Chapel Bridge Park
Newton, MA 02158
(617) 965-5200

Appendix 2: Vendors and Distributors

DU-IT Control Systems Group, Inc.
8765 Township Rd.
Shreve, OH 44676-9421
(216) 567-2906

Duxbury Systems
435 King St.
P.O. Box 1504
Littleton, MA 01460
(508) 486-9766

Edmark Corporation
P.O. Box 3903
Belleville, WA 98007
(800) 426-0856

EKEG Electronics Ltd.
P.O. Box 46199
Station G
Vancouver, BC, V6R 4G5
Canada
(604) 273-4358

E.M. VITU, Inc.
283 Peterson Rd.
Libertyville, IL 60048
(312) 367-4004

Enabling Technology
3102 S.E. Jay St.
Stuart, FL 34997
(407) 283-4817

Exceptional Parent Press
1170 Commonwealth Ave.
Boston, MA 02134
(617) 730-5800

Gallaudet University
800 Florida Ave, NE
Washington, D.C. 20002
(800) 672-6720

Harris Communications
Dept. GASK 9006
Minneapolis, MN 55408
(800) 825-6758 or (800) 825-9187 (TDD)

Henter-Joyce
7901 4th St, N.
Suite 211
St. Petersburg, FL 33702
(800) 969-5658

Hoolean Corp.
P.O. Box 230
Cornville, AZ 86325
(602) 634-7517

Howtek, Incorporated
21 Park Avenue
Hudson, NH 03051
(603) 882-5200

HumanWare
6245 King Rd.
Loomis, CA 95650
(800) 722-3393 or (916) 652-7253

IBM Education Systems National Support Center
P.O. Box 2150
Atlanta, GA 30055
(800) 426-2133 or (404) 988-2729 (TDD)

ILA (Independent Living Aids)
27 East Mall
Plainview, NY 11803
(800) 537-2118

Integrated Microcomputer Systems
2 Research Place
Rockville, MD 20850
(301) 948-4790 or (301) 869-6391 (TDD)

Itac Systems
3121 Benton Dr.
Garland, TX 75042
(800) 533-4822 or (214) 493-3073

Kinetic Designs
14231 Antevka Lane, SE
Ollal, WA 98466
(800) 453-0330 or (206) 857-7943

Krown Research
10371 West Jefferson Blvd.
Culver City, CA 90232
(800) 833-4968

Kurzweil Computer Products
185 Albany St.
Cambridge, MA 02139
(800) 343-0311 or (617) 864-4700

LC Technologies, Inc.
4415 Glen Rose St.
Fairfax, VA 22032
(800) 733-5284

L S & S Group
P.O. Box 673
Northbrook, IL 60065
(800) 468-4789 or (708) 498-9777

Luminaud Inc.
8688 Tyler Blvd.
Mentor, OH 44060
(216) 255-9082

MicroSpeed, Inc.
44000 Old Warmsprings Blvd.
Freemont, CA 94538
(415) 490-1403

Microsystems
600 Worcester Rd.
Suite B2
Framingham, MA 01701
(508) 626-8511

MicroTouch
10 State St.
Woburn, MA 01801
(617) 935-0081

NanoPac
4833 South Sheridan Rd.
Tulsa, OK 74145
(918) 665-0329

National Association of the Deaf
NAD Bookstore
814 Thayer Avenue
Silver Spring, MD 20910
(301) 587-6282

Newex, Inc.
695 DeLong Ave.
Novato, CA 94947
(415) 892-1573

Omnichron
1438 Oxford Ave.
Berkeley, CA 94709
(415) 540-6455

Optelec
4 Lyberty Way
Westford, MA 01886
(800) 828-1056 or (508) 393-0707

Personal Data Systems
100 West Rincon Ave.
Suite 217
P.O. Box 1008
Campbell, CA 95009
(408) 866-1126

Appendix 2: Vendors and Distributors 151

Personally Developed Software
P.O. Box 3266
Wallingford, CT 06492
(800) 426-7279

Phone TTY Inc.
202 Lexington Ave.
Hackensack, NJ 07601
(201) 489-7889 or (201) 489-7890
(TDD)

Pointer Systems
One Mill St.
Burlington, VT 05401
(800) 537-1562 or (802) 658-3260

Polytel Computer Products
1250 Oakmead Parkway
Suite 30
Sunnyvale, CA 94086
(800) 245-6655 or (408) 730-1347

Potomac Technology
1010 Rockville Pike, Suite 401
Rockville, MD 20852
(301) 762-4005 or (301) 762-0851
(TDD)

Prentke-Romich
1022 Heyl Rd.
Wooster, OH 44691
(800) 642-8255

ProHance Technologies
1307 S. Mary Ave. #104
Sunnyvale, CA 94087
(408) 746-0950

Radio Shack Division of Tandy
300 One Tandy Center
Fort Worth, TX 76102
(817) 390-3401

Raised Dots Computing
408 South Baldwin St.
Madison, WI 53703
(608) 257-9595

Regenesis Development Corp.
1046 Deep Cove Rd.
North Vancouver, BC V761S
Canada
(604) 929-6663

Seeing Technologies
7074 Brooklyn Blvd.
Minneapolis, MN 55429
(612) 560-8080

Services for Handicapped Persons
National Library of Canada
Ottawa, Ontario
K1A ON 4

Sign Media, Incorporated
Burtonsville Commerce Court
4020 Blackburn Lane
Burtonsville, MD 20866
(301) 421-0268

SoftLogic Solutions, Incorporated
One Perimeter Rd.
Manchester, NH 03103
(603) 627-9900

Street Electronics
6420 Via Real
Carpinteria, CA 93013
(805) 684-4593

Syntha-Voice Computers, Incorporated
125 Gailmont Dr.
Hamilton, Ontario,
Canada L8K4B8
(800) 263-4540
(416) 578-0565

Appendix 2: Vendors and Distributors

Talking Computer Systems
8 Riverside St. Suite 3-1
Watertown, MA 02172
(617) 926-1919

TASH Inc.
70 Gibson Dr.
UNH 12
Markham, ONT.
L3R 4C2 Canada
(416) 475-2212

Telecommunications for the Deaf, Inc.
814 Thayer Ave.
Silver Spring, MD 20910
(301) 589-3786 or (301) 589-3006 (TTD)

TeleSensory Products, Inc. (TSI)
455 N. Bernardo Ave.
P.O. Box 7455
Mt. View, CA 94039
(800) 969-9064

Toys For Special Children
385 Warburton Ave.
Hastings-on-Hudson, NY 10706
(914) 478-0960

Trace Center
S-151 Waisman Center
1500 Highland Ave.
Madison, WI 53705
(608) 262-6966

Trian Corp.
Suite 302
177 Telegraph Rd.
Bellingham, WA 98226

UltraTec
6442 Normandy Lane
Madison, WI 53719
(608) 273-0707

Versatron Corp.
103 Plaza St,
Healdsburg, CA 95488
(707) 433-8244

VIS-AIDS
102-09 Jamaica Ave.
Richmond Hills, NY 11418
(800) 346-9579 or (718) 847-4734

Visuaide 2000, Inc.
111 Rue St. Charles Ouest,
Tour Ouest
2E Etage, Longueuil, PQ
J4K 5G4 Canada
(514) 463-1717

Voice Connection Products
17835 Skypark Circle, Suite C
Irving, CA 92714
(714) 261-2366

Votrax Inc.
38455 Hills Tech Dr.
Farmington Hills, MI 48331
(313) 442-0900

Western Ctr. for Microcomputers Spec.
1259 El Camino Real, Suite 275
Menlo Park, CA 94025
(415) 326-6997

WesTest Engineering Corp.
1470 N. Main St.
Bountiful, UT 84010
(801) 289-7100

Windmills
C.G.C.E.D.P./EDD
P.O. Box 826880
MIC 41
Sacramento, CA 94280-0001

Xerox-Kurzweil Industries
185 Albany St.
Cambridge, MA 02139
(800) 343-0311

ZiCOM
2485-A Coral St.
Vista, CA 92083
(800) 621-5633
(619) 727-7110

ZYGO Industries
P.O. Box 1008
Portland, OR 97207-1008
(503) 684-6006

Appendix 3:
CD-ROM Titles that Translate into Special Format

*Note: An * denotes that the title translates with difficulty.*

About Cows

Bible Library

C CD-ROM

CD Music Guide

CD-ROM Sourcedisc 1990

CIA World Fact Book

Compton's Encyclopedia*

Computer Library

DISC Magazine

Facts on File News Digest

Grolier's Electronic Encyclopedia

Languages of the World

Library of the Future

McGraw-Hill Science and Technical Reference Set

Microsoft Bookshelf

Movie Database and Software Potpourri

PC-Blue

PDR*

Shareware Gold

U.S. History on CD-ROM

WordCruncher

World Almanac & Book of Facts

Appendix 4: Bulletin Boards Addressing Handicapped Person's Needs

*Note: An * denotes that although not a bulletin board, these online databases have the latest information on technological devices for the disabled.*

AbleData*
Newington Children's Hospital
c/o BRS a Division of Maxwell
8000 Westpark Dr.
McLean, VA 22102
(800) 289-4277

ADDS (Assistive Device Database System) American International Data Search, Inc.
650 University Ave.
Suite 101B
Sacramento, CA 95825
(916) 924-0280

Boston Computer Society
For further information and to set up your system call: (617) 767-2909

Committee on Personal Computers and the Handicapped (COPH-2)
2030 Irving Park Road
Chicago, IL 60618
(312) 477-1813
(312) 286-0608 (computer)

4-Sights Network
c/o Greater Association of Blind and Visually Impaired
16625 Grand River Ave.
Detroit, MI 48227
(313) 272-3900
(313) 272-7111 (computer)

Handicapped Educational Exchange (HEX)
11523 Charlton Drive
Silver Spring, MD 20902
(301) 681-7372
(301) 593-7033 (computer)

Handicapped Users Database
c/o Compuserve Information Service
5000 Arlington Center
Columbus, OH 43220
(800) 848-8990

IBM National Support Center Bulletin Board System (NSC-BBS). For further information and to set up your system call: (404) 835-5300

National Association of Blind and Visually Impaired Computer Users
P.O. Box 1352
Roseville, CA 95661
(916) 783-0364
(916) 786-3923 (computer)

SpecialWare Database *
LINC Resources, Inc.
4820 Indianola Avenue
Columbus, OH 43214
(614) 885-5599

Appendix 5:
Funding Sources for Adaptive Equipment

Private Corporations

The purchase of equipment for a library by a business benefits both. The business will realize a tax write-off for a charitable contribution and will receive positive public relations (if the library agrees to publicity). This approach may be most effective with a company that *needs* a boost in its image.

Trust Funds

Many people put part of their estate into a trust fund for a specific purpose. There may be one to assist people with disabilities in a bank in your area. Banks don't usually advertise this information however. To determine whether there are any such funds in your area, contact the trust division of each bank. Another source of information about funds is *The Foundation Directory* which lists funds and foundations. It can be found in large libraries. The larger foundations, such as the Ford Foundation, are typically inundated with requests, however, while local funds may sit untouched for years.

Alumni and Service Clubs

Local civic organizations such as Kiwanis, Rotary, Lions Club, and Alumni have often contributed to the purchase of equipment. Since funds are usually limited, it is best to use them sparingly and to suggest a "matching funds" arrangement with another source.

Fundraisers

Libraries often have affiliations with groups which may assist in a fundraising activity. "Friends" groups, coworkers, and other organizations (such as labor unions) have successfully raised funds by conducting raffles, bake sales, car washes, dinners, and other creative activities.

Public Appeals

If other sources of funding have been exhausted, a public appeal is an option. This form of funding procurement is not suggested as a regular avenue because people tend to become jaded if exposed to too many. It has proven to be a successful tactic in a number of cases and can serve to bring a community together.

Source: Carol Cohen, Consultant, Prentke-Romich Co.

Notes

Preface

1. The National Library Service (NLS) for the Blind was established in 1932 to serve as a vehicle to facilitate the circulation of braille to blind adults by having 19 libraries distribute books in braille format. Through various amendments, the NLS network is now comprised of 55 regional and 92 sub-regional libraries, serving all parts of the United States, Puerto Rico, the Virgin Islands and Guam. The network lends playback equipment, braille and recorded books to over 600,000 children and adults.

2. Recording for the Blind is a non-profit service organization that provides recorded educational books free on loan to individuals who cannnot read standard printed material because of a visual, physical or perceptual disabilty. *Recording for the Blind, Annual Report, 1989.*

3. It is believed that at one time or another every non-disabled person will be temporarily disabled for a short period of time. This temporary disability may be caused by something as harmless as an eye infection or as dramatic as a concussion lasting several weeks and preventing a person from accessing print information.

4. American Library Association, *ALA Handbook of Organizations* (1990/1991): 234-237.

Chapter 1

1. Trace Research and Development Center, "I Know Some Who Have a Disability. How Can A Computer Be Useful To Them?" *Trace Reprint Series, "Commonly Asked Questions"* (Madison, Wis.: University of Wisconsin, 1990).

2. Ibid.

3. Ibid.

4. Ibid.

5. Jerome Schein, "Do Ears Wear Out?" *The Voice* (September/October, 1990): 12.

6. The American Foundation for the Blind is a non-profit organization located in New York City. The foundation is home to the Sam S. Miguel Memorial Library (a library which has material on blindness), an assistive technology department and a planning and research department.

7. National Association for the Visually Impaired, "Why We Stand Alone," a position paper revised 8/1990.

8. Dana Bottorff, "Sales of Computers for the Disabled Suffer From Cost, Marketing Problems," *New England Business* (July 6, 1987): 24.

9. Joe Lazzaro, "Opening the Doors for the Disabled," *Byte* (August 1990): 258.

10. Ibid.

Chapter 2

1. Standard used by the National Library Service, U.S. Postal Authority, the National Association for the Visually Handicapped and most other organizations serving visually impaired persons.

Chapter 3

1. Harvey Laurer, "Why One Medium Isn't Enough," *OCLC Micro* 5, no. 6 (December 1989): 22.

2. Ibid.

3. Ibid.

4. Ibid., 23.

5. Ibid., 262.

6. A.M. Goldberg et al., "An Evaluation of Braille Translation Programs," *Journal of Visual Impairment and Blindness*. (December 1987): 490. When evaluated according to NLS standards (correct contractions, spelling, spacing, formatting PC Braille), scored an 88 out of 100.

7. Ibid. The Duxbury Translator scored a 92 in the NLS evaluation as the braille codes were properly applied and braille contractions observed.

8. The American Academy of Otolaryngology has determined that the sound level in a quiet library measures 30 decibels, 70 decibels of sound are measured in a busy traffic area or noisy restaurant and 90 decibels are heard in truck traffic or near a power mower. The noise level drops 6 decibels with

every doubling of distance from the source. A.M. Goldberg et al., "A Look at Six Printers," *Journal of Visual Impairment and Blindness* (June 1987): 276.

9. The height of the braille dot should be between .018 and .020 of an inch; the base diameter of each dot should be between .050-.065 of an inch; distance from center to center of adjacent dots in the same cell should be .092; distance in adjacent cells should be between .235 and .250 of an inch; distance from braille cells from line to line should not be less than .400 of an inch. Goldberg et al., "A Look at Six Printers," 272.

10. Ibid.

11. Ibid.

12. Ibid.

13. Ibid.

14. Ibid.

15. Ibid.

16. Phyllis Herrington and David Holladay, "The Ohtsuki Brailler," *Raised Dots Computing* (March/April 1990): 5.

17. Ibid.

18. Goldberg et al., "A Look at Six Printers," 278.

19. The consumers evaluating the braille found the spacing between the lines and cells good, but the height of the dots and consistency of the braille irregular. Goldberg et al., "A Look at Six Printers," 278.

20. Ibid.

21. Ibid., 284.

22. Ibid., 279.

23. Ibid.

24. Ibid., 280. It should also be noted that a Romeo printer used on a table during a meeting in a standard conference room of 20 x 15 ft. did not disturb either the speaker (who was able to continue to speak normally) nor those in attendance.

25. "Printer for the Blind," *Database Searcher* (April 1990): 34.

26. Barbara Wegreich, "The PC Is My Lifeline," *PC Computing* 2 (July 1989): 87.

162 Notes

Chapter 4

1. The original Kurzweil Reading Machine debuted on Walter Cronkite's News show in 1976 when it read aloud his sign-off message using synthetic speech. It weighed 350 pounds and cost over $50,000. Lawrence D. Maloney, "Raymond Kurzweil, Technical Visionary," *Design News* (February 12. 1990): 74-75.

2. A. Meyers and E. Schreier, "An Evaluation of Speech Access Programs," *Journal of Visual Impairment and Blindness* (January 1990): 26.

3. Ibid.

4. Ibid., and *Second Beginner's Guide to Personal Computers for the Blind and Visually Impaired*, (Boston: National Braille Press, 1987).

5. Jim Turri and Curtis Chong, "Artic Vision," in *Second Beginner's Guide to Personal Computers*, 67, 72.

6. Several commands in the program require the users not using the Gizmo to actually lift their right hand from the home keys to depress keys—impossible for some physically handicapped, challenging for some visually impaired without braille orientation keytops. Meyers and Schreier, "Evaluation," 35; Turri and Chong, "Artic Vision," 72.

7. Both manual and instructions contain keyboard orientation. Meyers and Schreier, "Evaluation," 27.

8. Ibid.

9. Screen access programs evaluated (using the criteria of reading all material from the screen, editing, compatibility, reading ability and ease of installation) were Flipper, HAL, JAWS, IBM Screen Reader, SpeaquaLizer, Vert-Plus and Visions. Ibid., 30.

10. Ibid., 31.

11. Paul Filpus, "A Better Screen Reader," *Dialogue With The Blind* (Fall 1990): 47.

12. Meyers and Schreier, "Evaluation," 32.

13. Ibid.

14. A way around the problem of needing "computer literacy" to use this program is to have a tech person make a boot disk for every application.

15. With the exception of Artic's SynPhonix synthesizer, this listing was compiled by IBM's National Support Center For Persons With Disabilities,

because all will work with the IBM Screen Reader. The listing was not intended as an endorsement for warranty purposes with the Screen Reader.

16. Joe Lazzaro, "Talking Networks, Computers That Speak While Talking To Each Other," *LAN Magazine* (August 1990): 137.

17. Slimware, a good driver priced at $600, will only drive the Syntha-Voice synthesizers. It has a "sticky key" feature which allows a physically impaired person to group a series of multiple keystrokes together. It is available from Syntha-Voice Computers.

18. HAL (short for Haled) is a standard software driver developed by Dolphin Industries of Worcester, England and distributed by BIT Technologies. It has two modes: "read" which allows the user to change the pitch and speed and has a notepad for users; and "live" which allows the user to develop up to 10 user windows. Meyers and Schreier, "Evaluation," 28-29.

Chapter 5

1. L. Converso and S. Hocek, "Optical Character Recognition," *Journal of Visual Impairment and Blindness* (December 1990).

2. M.M. Usla et al., "A Review of Optical Character Recognition Systems," *Journal of Visual Impairment and Blindness* (May 1990): 221.

3. Basically, all this involves is opening the computer's chassis, slipping the card in an open slot, reconfiguring the system if necessary and following a step-by-step software installation.

4. Usla et al., "A Review," 223.

5. Bruce Brown, "Supercharging Your Scanner," *PC Magazine* (March 28, 1989).

6. Usla et al., "A Review," 223.

7. Contact Xerox-Kurzweil for further information.

8. Usla et al., "A Review," 222.

9. John Webster, "Personal Reader Changes Written Words to Speech" (Documents Are Converted to Speech Using Kurzweil Computer Products' Personal Reader), *PC Week* (October 10, 1988): 17.

10. "Lion's Club KPR Donations Making a Difference For Communities," *Xerox-Kurzweil Personal Reader Update* (Winter/Spring 1990): 1.

11. Fareed Haj, "From Scanner to Braille Through Teamwork" and "Producing Braille by Scanning," *Raised Dots Computing* (March/April, May/June 1990): 5-12.

Chapter 6

1. Milton Blackstone, "What's the Big Idea?" (Voice-Activated Computer Technology for the Handicapped), *Mainstream* (November 1989): 31.

2. IBM, *Resource Guide for Persons With Mobility Impairments* (August 1990): 5.

3. A copy of Encore.COM source code, developed by Scott Chaney, is available from *PC Magazine*, by sending your name, address and postcard to: PC Magazine, One Park Avenue, New York, NY 10016; Attn: Katherine West. Scott Chaney, "Automate Your Program Operations With Encore.COM," *PC Magazine* (April 16, 1991): 327-335.

4. Activation pressure for keys to be activated is measured in ounces or grams for this discussion. If you would like a better understanding of this measurement, press downward on a kitchen scale with one finger and you will see the marker move from ounce to ounce.

Chapter 7

1. "Power Mouse Courts 1-2-3- Users," *Byte* 1 (12) (November 1989): 220.

2. "Mice and Trackballs: Choices for the New Generation of Applications; Prochance Technologies Power Mouse 100" (one of 32 evaluations of alternate input devices), *PC Magazine* (August 1990): 268.

3. Blackstone, "Big Idea," 31.

4. Rehabilitation dollars are still in short supply, which means that an "able-minded" person who survived catastrophic trauma may not have gotten all the training needed to return to the learning environment. As one technician related, "insurance dollars are poured into hospital care to keep the individual from dying, but there are no dollars to help this person return to the accepted norm (i.e., jobs, access technology)."

5. For further information on sources and types of switches to access computers please see *Resource Guide for Mobility Impairment*, 43-46. Product catalogs for TASH and ZYCO provide an excellent overview of all switches and are available free of charge.

6. John Webster, "Reflector Technology Frees the Disabled to Move Cursor With a Nod of The Head," *PC Week* (July 4, 1988): 17.

7. IBM, "Technology For Persons with Disabilities; An Introduction," August 1990, 4.

8. David Bayer, Rick Nash and John Sprinsteen, "Design Philosophy for LIASON by DU-It Control Systems Group," Paper, October 1988, 1.

9. President's Committee on Employment of People With Disabilities, "New DragonDictate Computer Software Turns Headset Into a Keyboard," *Worklife* (Summer 1990): 11

10. Ibid.

11. Dr. Salyers related the story of Herbert Hoffman, a professional with severe Cerebral Palsy who lived in Chicago and worked for the U.S. Weather Service. Dr. Salyers, who rehabilitated many people with Cerebral Palsy, said he could not understand him. But DragonDictate, after listening to the young man for two hours, was able to learn his words, obey his commands and speak to or for him. Since DragonDictate was correct 85 percent of the time this gentleman with Cerebral Palsy has a good and meaningful job. President's Committee, "DragonDictate," 11.

12. IBM, "Technology," 91.

13. Ibid., 92.

14. Blackstone, "Big Idea," 31; IBM, "Technology," 69.

Chapter 8

1. Susan Cohen, "TDD Access in Public Libraries: 15 Years Later," *Interface* (Summer 1990): 11.

2. "Senator Simon's Office Installs TDD" and "About the IBM PhoneCommunicator," *GA-SK Newsletter* (Winter 1990): 6.

3. IBM, *Resource Guide for Persons with Hearing Impairments* (August 1990): 11, 12.

4. Sandra Edwards, "Computer Technology: Breakthroughs for the Hearing and Speech Impaired," *OCLC Micro* (August 1990): 29.

Chapter 9

1. Maggie Bacon of the State Library of Michigan estimates that it takes one 45-minute session to orient a new computer user to the keyboard, speech

device and the various screen setups. It takes an additional five hours to train a person in Boolean search techniques. If the user does find print material he wants, the material is retrieved and he is instructed on the mechanics of the Kurzweil Personal Reader.

2. Maria Witt, "The Online Public Access Catalogue at the Cite des Sciences Mediatheque in Paris," *Electronic Library* (February 1990): 36-44.

3. Lazzaro, "Talking Networks," *LAN Magazine*, 138-39.

4. David Holladay, "CD-ROM Technology is Here," *Raised Dots Computing Newsletter* (January/February 1991): 3.

5. Anita Richaume, "How Blind People Access Data Stored on CD-ROM in University Libraries," Paper presented at the IFLA General Conference and council Meeting, Division of Libraries Serving the General Public, Section of Libraries for the Blind, Paris, France, 1989.

6. Lazzaro, "Talking Networks," *LAN Magazine,* 138; Dave Holladay, "CD-ROM Technology," *Raised Dots,* 7.

7. Herb Brody, "The Great Equalizer—PC's Empower the Disabled," *PC Computing*, Ziff-Davis Publishing, CD-ROM edition, "Health Resources Library."

8. These users include: Lisa Davis, Iowa Regional Library, Judith Dixon, David Holladay, Joe Lazzaro and Barbara Mates.

9. Mary Roatch, "Accessibility Issues Addressed At PLA's Very Best Workshops II," *Interface* (Summer 1990): 13.

10. Project EASI, "Computers and Students with Disabilities: New Challenges for Higher Education," Project of the EDUCOM Educational Uses of Technology, September 1989, 9.

11. Ibid.

12. Sonita Cummings, "For Vision Impaired Patrons," (Ready Reference Methods that Work—a column), *Library Journal* (May 15, 1990): 23.

13. Jack Moore, "Finding the Right Educational Software For Your Child," *Exceptional Parent* (October, 1990): 59-62.

14. University at Buffalo, State University of Buffalo, "Health Sciences Library Services For Persons With Disabilities," Policy Statement [n.d.]: 1.

15. The ASCLA, division of the ALA, Academic Librarians Assisting the Disabled Discussion Group, has determined by an informal call for policy statements that the following institutions have working documents: Auraria Higher Education Center (Denver, Colorado), Columbia University, San Jose

State University Library, University at Buffalo, and the University of Kansas. Copies of the statements can be obtained by writing to: Current Chair, c/o ALA, ASCLA, Academic Librarians Assisting the Disabled Discussion Group, 50 East Huron Street, Chicago, Illinois 60611.

16. Ruth Velleman, *Meeting the Needs of People with Disabilities* (Phoenix, AZ: Oryx Press, 1990), 13-14. Ohio Library Association, Outreach and Special Services Division, Barbara Mates, General Editor, Brochure Series on Service Guidelines to Special Populations, December 1990.

Chapter 10

1. Carol Lea Clark, "Computer Technology: Hands-On Accessibility—Computer Equipment for the Disabled," *Arthritis Today* (November/December 1990): 26.

2. "High-Tech Aids Offer New Options to Deaf, Blind," *Futurist* (September/October 1989): 50.

3. Diana Prufer and Bill Shapiro, "Miracles in the Making," *Parenting* (December/January 1991): 27-28.

4. James Smith, "VA to Test PC System for the Handicapped" (Veteran Affairs Department's 30-day Evaluation of the Eyegaze System), *Government Computer News* 9, no. 6: 114. Copyright Ziff-Davis Publishing.

5. "Braille Mouse (Model II)," *Research and Development* (October 1989): 69.

6. Ellliot Schreier, "The Future of Access Technology for the Blind and Visually Impaired People," *Journal of Visual Impairment and Blindness* (December 1990): 522.

7. Americans with Disabilities Act of 1990, Public Law 101-336, 42 USC 12101-12213, Section 2 (2-8), discussed by Michael G. Gunde in "What Every Librarian Should Know About the ADA of 1990," *American Libraries* 22, no.8 (September 1991): 806-809.

8. Ibid., section 101(1) and section 106.

9. Ibid., sections 201 (2), 202.

10. Ibid., sections 301 (9); 302 (a); 302 (b)(1)(A); 302 (b)(1) (B); Section 302 (b)(2)(A).

11. Monica Frangini, "Tools for IBM PS/2 are Helpful for Overcoming Disabilities" (IBM Canada honored for sponsoring Research), *Computing Canada* (November 23, 1989): 24.

Glossary

Adaptive Technology Devices A wide variety of electronic items which enable an even wider variety of people with disabilities to live independently. Many of the devices are based on computer technology.

ASCII American Standard Code for Information Interchange. A standard set of characters used by computers. There are 128 ASCII characters. This "universal language" allows adaptive technology to work.

Board An integrated circuit board which plugs into a slot (open space) in the computer.

Boot To turn on or restart a computer.

Braille A writing system using raised dots in a pattern (cell) which represents the standard Arabic alphabet.

Braille Embosser/Printer A device which produces braille mechanically or electronically; some are driven by a PC.

Card See **Board**

Carriage Length The maximum number of characters on a line varies with type of print used.

Closed Captioning A method by which American Sign Language translations are either broadcast live to television sets with captioning decoders or laid down on a track of videotape recordings. This allows the hearing impaired or deaf person to hear the dialogue as it is being spoken.

Closed Circuit Display (CCD) A closed circuit system which enlarges almost any item placed on its viewing tray.

Closed Circuit TV (CCTV) A system consisting of a television camera which takes a picture of an item and projects the enlarged display on a monitor.

Expanded Keyboard Keys are larger and are configured to enable a person with limited strength and dexterity to lightly tap information into the computer.

170 Glossary

Grade II Braille This is the accepted form of written braille communication. It consists of the braille alphabet, numbers and punctuation marks in an abbreviated format. Common words and letter contractions are reduced to a type of shorthand which eliminates the need to spell out frequently used words like "with" or "the" and eliminates the tedium of printing and reading a cell for every letter.

Head-Pointer The optical light-beam pointers select from a keyboard displayed on the screen.

Interface Card See **Switch Interface**.

Large Print A print type which is larger than 13.9.

Large-Print Screen Displays This takes on many formats, which can be a simple magnifier, closed television-type technology or an enlarged screen.

Membrane Keyboard This is a flat keyboard—keys are not raised.

Menu A programming technique which lists choices that are available to the user to select from.

Micro-Keyboard A keyboard on which the keys are grouped as closely together as possible so fingers that cannot stretch over the rows do not have to.

Mouthstick A mouthpiece which serves as a "finger" to control a computer (or other device). The user is able to manipulate the controls using this small device.

OCR Scanner A computer-based optical character recognition system that translates material into an electronic format that can then be stored and accessed via a computer monitor, a printer or an adapted device such as a speech synthesizer or braille display.

Paperless Braille A device which translates the ASCII notations it sees to small pins that are raised or lowered electronically to form different braille characters.

Phoneme One of the smallest units of speech that serve to distinguish one utterance from another.

Refreshable Braille A changeable braille display; no "hard copy" is made.

Glossary 171

Screen Reader A software program, used with a speech synthesizer, to properly interpret and read.

Speech Synthesizer A device which reads aloud material found on computer screens, a screen reader must be used with it to tell it how to read the material.

Switch Interface A software or hardware device which acts as a link between the switch and the computer.

Switches These are used in conjunction with a hardware or software device providing input to the computer.

Synthesizer An artificial voice which translates written ASCII text into artificial voice output.

TDD Telecommunications Devices for the Deaf is a device which allows hearing and speech impaired individuals as well as deaf persons to access the phone lines and communicate with each other and the non-impaired user. The users type messages back and forth instead of talking into a receiver.

Trace Center Was founded in 1971 to address the communication needs of people who are non-speaking and have severe disabilities. It has evolved over the years and now focuses on: communication (i.e., how non-speaking and physically impaired people can converse using high-technology communications aids); control (developing control mechanisms for computers and living aids); and computer access (ways to make all computers more accessible to people with disabilities).

Voice Recognition A device which is programmed to recognize the voice of the user and execute the voice commands made by the user.

Bibliography

Books and Articles

"About the IBM PhoneCommunicator." *GA/SK* 22, no.1 (Winter 1990).
American Association of Retired Persons. "A Profile of Older Americans." Washington: American Association of Retired Persons, 1989.
———. "Truth About Aging: Guidelines for Accurate Communications" Washington: American Association of Retired Persons, 1986.
American Foundation for the Blind. *Directory of Services for Blind and Visually Impaired Persons in the United States.* 23d. ed. New York: American Foundation for the Blind, 1988.
———. "How Does a Blind Person Get Around?" New York: American Foundation for the Blind, 1970.
———. "What To Do When You Meet a Deaf-Blind Person." New York: American Foundation for the Blind, 1986.
American Foundation for the Blind and Visually Impaired Persons, National Tech Center. *Sources of Products for the Blind and Visually Impaired.* New York: AFB, 1990.
American Library Association. *ALA Handbook of Organization, 1990/1991.* Chicago: American Library Association, 1990.
Arthritis Foundation. "Basic Facts: Answers to Your Questions." Atlanta, GA: Arthritis Foundation, 1989.
Balas, Janet. "Seniornet: Computer Skills for Senior Citizens." *Computers in Libraries* 9, no. 8 (Sept. 1989): 24-26.
Baskin, Barbara H., and Karen H. Harris. *The Mainstreamed Library: Issues, Ideas, Innovations.* Chicago: American Library Association, 1982.
Bayer, David, and John Springsteen. "Design Philosophy for LIAISON by DU-IT." Unpublished paper, 1988.
Blackstone, Milton. "What's the Big Idea?" *Exploding Myths.* 14 (Nov. 1989).
Bottorff, Dana. "Sales of Computers for Disabled Suffer From Cost, Marketing Problems." *New England Business Journal*, 9 (July 6, 1987).
Brightman, A. "Challenging the Myth of Disability." *EDUCOM Review 1989* 24, no. 4 (Winter 1989): 17-23.
Brody, Herb. "The Great Equalizer-PC's Empower the Disabled." *PC Computing*, Ziff-Davis Publishing, CD-ROM ed. July 1989.
Brown, Bruce. "Supercharging Your Scanner." *PC Magazine* 8, no.6 (March 28, 1989).

Bruhn, Suzanne. "The Provision of Library Services For People With Disabilities: An Incentive to Change?" *The Australian Library Journal* 38 (May 1989): 133-140.

Center for Special Education Technology. *Assistive Technology Resource Directory*. Reston, VA: Center for Special Education Technology, 1990.

Chaney, Scott. "Automate Your Program Operations With Encore.Com." *PC Magazine* 10, no.7 (April 16, 1991).

Clark, Carol Lea. "Computer Technology: Hands On Accessibility." *Arthritis Today*, 4 (Nov./Dec. 1990).

Closing the Gap. *Closing the Gap Resource Directory: A Guide to Selection of Microcomputer Technology* Henderson: MN: Closing the Gap, 1989.

Cohen, Susan. "TDD Access in Libraries: 15 Years Later." *Interface* 12, no.4 (Summer 1990).

Computers for the Hearing Impaired, January 1977-October, 1989: A Bibliography. Springfield, VA: National Technical Information Service. Pub. no: PB 90-8560249/HCW. 1989.

Converso, L., and S. Hocek. "Optical Character Recognition."*Journal of Visual Impairment and Blindness*. 84, no.10 (Dec. 1990).

Cummings, Sonita. "For Vision Impaired Patrons," (Ready Reference Methods that Work—a column), *Library Journal*. 115 (May 15, 1990).

Dixon, Judith M. and Jane Mandelbaum. "Reading Through Technology: Evolving Methods and Opportunities for Print-Handicapped Individuals." *Journal of Visual Impairment and Blindness*. 84, no. 10 (Dec. 1990): 493-96.

Edwards, Sandra. "Computer Technology: Breakthroughs for the Hearing and Speech Impaired." *OCLC Micro* 6, no.4 (Aug. 1990).

———. "Computer Technology and the Physically Disabled." *OCLC Micro* 5, no.6 (Dec. 1989).

———. "Microcomputers and the Visually Impaired" (Low-Vision to No-Vision). *OCLC Micro* 5, no.6 (Dec. 1989).

Eldridge, L. *R is for Reading: Library Service to Blind and Physically Handicapped Children*. Washington, D.C.: National Library Service for the Blind and Physically Handicapped, 1985.

Ellefson, Mary Ann, and Don Ellefson. *When You Meet a Person in a Wheelchair*. Minneapolis: Sister Kenny Institute, 1983.

Enders, Alexandra, ed. *Assistive Technology Sourcebook*. Washington, D.C.: RESNA, 1989.

———. *Funding for Assistive Technology and Related Services: An Annotated Bibliography*. Washington, D.C.: Electronic Industries Foundation, Rehabilitation Engineering Center, 1989.

ERIC Clearinghouse on Handicapped and Gifted Children. "Being At Ease With Handicapped Children: ERIC Digest." Reston, VA: Council for Exception Children. 2 page brochure.

Filpus, Paul. "A Better Screen Reader." *Dialogue With the Blind* 29, no.1 (1990): 46-50.

Frangini, Monica. "Tools for IBM PS/2 Are Helpful for Overcoming Disabilities." *Computing Canada* (Nov. 23, 1989).

Furlong, Mary, and Greg Kearsley. "Computer Instruction for Older Adults." *Generations* 11, no. 1 (Fall 1986): 32-35.

Gacioch, Marti, and Dennis Wool. "Chips Ahoy! Computer Systems for Physically Disabled." *Mainstream* 15 (August 1990): 19-27.

Gething, Lindsay, and Rosemary Leonard, and Kate O'Loughlin. *Person to Person: Community Awareness of Disability.* Sydney, Austrailia: MacLennan & Petty, 1989.

Gold, Peter S. "CD-ROM for the Development of Low Vision Technology." *CD-Rom EndUser* 2, no. 1 (May 1990): 36-37.

Goldberg, A.M., E. Schreir, J.D. Levanthal, and J.C. DeWitt. "An Evaluation of Braille Translation Programs." *Journal of Visual Impairment and Blindness.* 81, no.10 (Dec. 1987).

———. "A Look at Six Printers." *Journal of Visual Impairment and Blindness.* 81, no.6 (June 1987).

Greenblatt, Susan L., ed. *Providing Services for People With Vision Loss: A Multidisciplinary Perspective.* Lexington, MA: Resources for Rehabilitation, 1989.

Gunde, Michael G. "What Every Librarian Should Know About the ADA of 1990." *American Libraries* 22, no.8 (September 1991): 806-809.

Haj, Faheed. "From Scanner to Braille Through Teamwork." *Raised Dots Computing Newsletter* 8, no.83 (March/April 1990).

———. "Producing Braille by Scanning." *Raised Dots Computing Newsletter* 8, no.84 (May/June 1990).

Herrington, Phyllis, and David Holladay. "The Ohtsuki Brailler." *Raised Dots Computing Newsletter* 8, no. 83 (March/April 1990).

Hoffman, Ann. *Many Faces of Funding.* Mill Valley, CA: Phonic Ear, 1990.

Holladay, David. "CD-ROM Technology Is Here." *Raised Dots Computing Newsletter* 9, no.88 (Jan./Feb, 1991).

IBM National Support Center for Persons With Disabilities, Atlanta: GA: IBM, 1990: "Technology for Persons With Disabilities: An Introduction"; "Resource Guide for Persons With Hearing Impairments"; "Resource Guide for Persons With Learning Impairments"; "Resource Guide for Persons With Mobility Impairments"; "Resource Guide for Persons With Vision Impairments."

Klauber, Julie. "What Do They Do When They See a Blind Person?": tips for sensitizing library staff. *Library Outreach Reporter* 3 (Spring 1990): 34-35.

Lang, Jovian P. *Unequal Access to Information; Resources, Problems and Needs of the World's Information Poor.* Ann Arbor, MI: Pierian Press, 1988.

Lauer, Harvey. "Why One Medium Isn't Enough." *OCLC Micro* 5, no.6 (Dec. 1989).

Lazzaro, Joe. "Opening Doors for the Disabled." *BYTE* 15, no.16 (Aug. 1990).

―――. "Talking Newtworks, Computers That Speak Whiile Talking to Each Other." *LAN Magazine* 5, no.8 (August 1990).

Lee, Kai-Fu, and Alexander G. Hauptman, and Alexander I. Rudnicky. "The Spoken Word." *BYTE* 15, no. 7 (July 1990): 225-32.

Library of Michigan, Service for the Blind and Physically Handicapped. "Handicapped Work Station Now Available." *Prespective* 7, no. 1, 1989.

Lovejoy, Eunice G. *Portraits of Library Service to People With Disabilities.* Boston: G.K. Hall, 1989.

McCarty, Lyle. "Special Alloy is Key to Braille Display." *Design News* 29, no.1 (Feb. 12, 1990).

Maloney, Lawrence D. "Raymond Kurzweil Technical Visionary." *Design News* 29, no.1 (Feb. 12, 1990).

Mates, Barbara. "CD-ROM: A New Light for the Blind and Visually Impaired." *Computers in Libraries* (March 1990): 17-20.

―――. "More Light for the Blind" (Sidebar article discussing use of Search CD450 by the visually impaired computer user). *OCLC Micro* 6, no. 5 (Oct. 1990): 36.

Meyers, A., and E. Schreier. "An Evaluation of Speech Access Programs." *Journal of Viusal Impairment and Blindness* 84, no.1 (Jan. 1990).

"Mice & Trackballs: Choices for the New Generation." *PC Magazine* 9, no.14 (Aug. 1990).

Moore, Jack. "Finding the Right Educational Software for Your Child." *Exceptional Parent* 28, no.7 (Oct. 1990).

National Association for the Visually Impaired. "Why We Stand Alone." A position paper, revised 8/1990.

National Association of the Deaf. "Some Information About People With Hearing Impairments." Silver Spring, MD: National Association of the Deaf. [n.d.].

National Braille Press. *Second Beginner's Guide to Personal Computers for the Blind and Visually Impaired.* Boston: National Braille Press, 1987.

National Easter Seal Society. *Myths and Facts about People Who Have Disabilities.* Chicago: National Easter Seal Society, 1986.

National Library Service for the Blind and Physically Handicapped. *Blindness and Visual Impairments: National Information and Advocacy Organizations.* 1990.

———. *Building a Library Collection on Blindness and Physical Disabilities: Basic Materials and Resources.* December, 1990.

———. "Computer Technology for Handicapped Persons." Fact Series, 1987.

———. *Library Resources for the Blind and Physically Handicapped.* Washington, D.C.: Library of Congress, 1989.

———. *National Organizations Concerned with Visually and Physically Handicapped Persons.* 1983.

———. *Reading, Writing, and Other Communication Aids for Visually and Physically Handicapped Persons.* 1986.

———. *Sources of Audiovisual Materials About Handicapping Conditions.* 1985.

———. *That All May Read, Library Service for the Blind and Physically Handicapped.* Washington, D.C.: Library of Congress, 1983.

Ohio Library Association pamphlet series, Barbara Mates, gen. ed. *Serving the Senior Library Patron, Serving the Severely Mentally Disabled Library Patron, Serving the Blind or Visually Impaired Library Patron, Serving the Deaf and Hearing Impaired Library Patron, Serving the Orthopedically Impaired Library Patron, Serving the Dyslexic and Learning Disabled Library Patron,* and *Serving the Chemically Dependent Library Patron.* Columbus, OH: Ohio Library Association, Outreach & Special Services Division, 1990.

Park, Leslie. *How to be a Friend to the Handicapped: A Handbook and Guide.* New York: Vantage Press, 1987.

"Power Mouse Courts 1-2-3 Users." *BYTE* 14, no.4 (Nov. 1989).

President's Committee on Employment of People With Disabilities. "Learning Disability: Not Just a Problem Children Outgrow." Washington, D.C.: President's Committee on Employment of People With Disabilities, 1989.

———. "New Dragon Dictate Computer Software Turns Headset Into A Keyboard." *Worklife* 3, no.2 (Summer 1990).

"Printer for the Blind." *Database Searcher* 6, no.4 (April 1990).

Project EASI. "Computers and Students with Disabilities: New Challenges for Higher Education." *Project of EDUCOM* (Sept. 1989).

Prufer, Diana, and Bill Shapiro. "Miracles in the Making." *Parenting* (Dec./Jan. 1991): 127-34.

Recording for the Blind. *1989 Annual Report Recording for the Blind.*
Research & Development 100. "Braille Mouse II." *Research and Development.* 31, no.10 (Oct. 1989): 69.
Richaume, Anita. "How Blind People Access Data Stored on CD-ROM in University Libraries." Paper presented at the IFLA General Conference & Council Meeting, Divisions of Libraries Serving the Public, Section of Libraries for the Blind, Paris, France, 1989.
Sandhu, Jim Singh, and Steve Richardson. *Concerned Technology, 1989: Electronic Aids for People With Special Needs.* Newcastle Upon Tyne Polytechnic, Handicapped Persons Research Unit, 1988.
Schein, Jerome. "Do Ears Wear Out?" *The Voice* 6, no.4 (Sept./Oct. 1990).
Schreier, Elliot. "The Future of Access Technology for Blind and Visually Impaired People." *Journal of Visual Impairment and Blindness* 84, no.10 (Dec. 1990).
"Senator Simon's Office Installs TDD." *GA/SK* 22, no.1 (Winter 1990).
Smith, James. "VA to Test PC System for the Handicapped" (Veteran Affairs Department's 30-day Evaluation of the Eyegaze System). *Government Computer News.* Copyright Ziff-Davis Publishing, Vol. 9, no. 6.
Smithsonian News Service. "High-Tech Aids Offer New Options to Deaf, Blind." *Futurist.* 23 (Sept./Oct. 1989): 50-51.
Telecommunications for the Deaf. "GA-SK Newsletter." 21, no.3 (Summer 1990).
"Tips You Can Use When Communicating With Deaf People." Rochester NY: National Technical Institute for the Deaf, 1983.
Trace Research & Development Center. "I Know Someone Who Has A Disability, How Can A Computer be Useful to Them?" *Trace Reprint Series, "Commonly Asked Qustions,"* (Jan. 1990).
Tweed, Prudence K., and Jason C. Tweed. *Colleges That Enable: A Guide to Support Services Offered to Physically Disabled Students on 40 U.S. Campuses.* Oil City, PA: Park Avenue Press, 1989.
University of Buffalo, Policy Statement. "Health Sciences Library Services for Persons With Disabilities." Buffalo, NY [n.d.], 1.
Uslan, M.M., E.M. Schrier, J.D. Levanthal, and A. Meyers. "A Review of Optical Recognition Systems." *Journal of Visual Impairment and Blindness* 84, no.5 (May 1990).
Vanderheiden, Gregg, et al., eds. *Trace Resourcebook: Assistive Technologies for Communication, Control, and Computer Access.* Madison, WI: Trace Reasearch and Development Center, University of Wisonsin, 1989.
Velleman, Ruth A. *Meeting the Needs of People with Disabilities; a Guide for Librarians, Educators and Other Service Professionals.* Phoenix, AZ: Oryx, 1990.

Voedisch, Ginni. "Librarianability-Access For All." *OCLC Micro* 6, no. 5 (Oct. 1990): 32-39.

Webster, John. "Personal Reader Changes Written Words to Speech." *PC Week* 5, no.41 (Oct. 1988).

———. "Reflector Technology Frees the Disabled To Move Cursor With A Nod of the Head." *PC Week* 5, no.27 (July 4, 1988).

Wegreich, Barbara. "The PC is My Lifeline." *PC Computing* (July 1989).

Witt, Maria. "The Online Public Access Catalogue at the Cite des Sciences Mediatheque in Paris." *Electronic Library* (Feb. 1990).

Wright, Keith, and Judith F. Davie. *The Library Manager's Guide to Hiring and Serving Disabled Persons.* Jefferson, NC: McFarland & Co., 1990.

Xerox-Kurzweil. "Lions Club KPR Donations Making a Difference in Communities." *Xerox-Kurzweil Personal Reader Update* 2, no.1 (Winter/Spring 1990).

Ziss, Audrey. "Disability Is a Myth: Technology = Liberation for Even the Most Profoundly Impaired." *Collegiate Microcomputer* 8, no.2 (May 1990): 155-58.

Videos

"A Place Where I Belong." Serving Disabled Children in the Library. 16 min. Available from: Services for Handicapped Persons, National Library of Canada.

"Have You Heard About the Deaf?" 34 min. Available from National Association of the Deaf.

"I Should Know A Lot, I Been Around So Long." Stories of Persons With Mental Retardation Who Have Lived Long Lives. 27 min. Available from: Exceptional Parent Press.

"People First." Serving and Employing People With Disabilities. 38 min. Available from: ALA Video.

"Windmills." A 14-hour modular training program developed by the California Governor's Committee for Employment of Disabled Persons. Available from Windmills.

Consult *Sources of Audiovisual Materials about Handicapping Conditions* (National Library Service for the Blind and Physically Handicapped) for further suggestions.

General Index

ACCESS, project, 127
Aging population, 4-7
Air cushion switch. *See* Switches, and mouth control
American Congress of the Blind, 27
American Foundation for the Blind, 7, 40, 44, 49, 64-65, 140, 160
American Library Association, Bill of Rights, xi
Americans With Disabilities Act (ADA), 115, 140-142
Audio-output, definition, 47-9. *See also* Synthesizers

Blindness and accessing information, 2, 45-46, 126, 128
  audio access, 47-62
  braille access, 27-46
Blindness
  definition of, 3
  statistics, 3-6, 145
Boston Public Library, 127
Braille
  computer produced, 2, 33-45, 161
  definition of, 169
  embossers, 40-45
  hardware translators, 32-33, 39
  keyboard and key indicators, 28-29
  mouse, 139-40
  need for, 8, 27-28, 46
  printers, *see* Embossers
  screen readers, *see* Paperless braille display

  software translators, 1-2, 33-39
  thermal jet printing, 45-46

Calera Recognition Systems, 64-65
California Community College system, 128
Canada, libraries, 133, 151
  Bloorview, 147
  Designing Aids for Disabled Adults (DADA), 148
  EKEG Electronics Ltd., 149
  Regnesis Development Corp., 151
  Services for Handicapped Persons, 151
  Syntha-Voice Computers, Inc., 151
  TASH, 152
  VISUAIDE 2000, Inc., 152
CCD/CCTV, 20-24
CD-ROM
  general configurations for, 117-18
  large-print access, 118-121
  audio access, 121-123
  braille access, 29, 124-25
  need for alternative media output, x, 10, 116
  potential problems, 123
  systems, 130-31
  titles which will translate, 124, 154
Chester County Public Library, 129
Cleveland Public Library, xi, 9, 116
Closed captioning
  definition, 112

growth, 112-13
and law, 112
productions with, 113
Collection development, 124, 131-32, 154
Commercial vendors of adaptive devices, 146-153

Deaf, statistics, 7
Deaf and communication, 107
computers, 110-11, 126
in-person, 113-14
telephone, *see* TTD/TTY
voice mail translators, 111
Deaf/blind
computer access and, 139
needs, 28
Deafnet, 111
Deaftek, 111
Disk guides, 73-74
Dynamic braille. *See* Paperless braille display
Dyslexia and Computers. *See* Learning disabled

Embossers, 40-45

Financing adaptive equipment, 129, 157
Florida Regional Library for the Blind, 128
Font selection and large print, 24-25
Foot control for entry, 85
Furniture selection for accessibility, 83

Guidelines to service for disabled, 134, 166-67

Head control for entry. *See* Switches, and head control
Hearing impairment, statistics, 6-7

Interface card, need for, 85-87
Interfaces, for special entry
CINTEX, 86;
DaDa entry, 87;
joysticks, 83-84, 94;
LIAISON, 99;
scanning devices, 96-97;
switches, 88-95
voice, 101-04

Keller, Helen, 28
Key sequencing. *See* Keystroke reduction
Keyboard
configurations, 81
emulators, 99, *see also* Switches; Voice input
expanded, 75-79
interfaces, 85-87
membrane, 2, 74-77, 88
reprogramming, 74-81
smaller, 2, 79-81
Keylocks, hardware, 73
Keystroke reduction, 71
hardware solutions, 76-81
software solutions, 71-72
Kurzweil, Raymond, 47, 63, 162

Language disorders, computer aid for, 1, 103-05, 125, 165
Large print
definition, 11, 160
hardcopy, 24-25
keytops, 12
need for, 8, 11-12
screen displays
hardware solution, 19
software solution, 13-18
styles of, 24
TDD/TTY's, 110
LEAP (Library Equal Access Project. *See* Seattle Public Library

Learning disabled, 1, 125. *See also* Audio-output
Libraries providing access to disabled
  Canada, 133
  France, 115, 116
  United States, 67, 115-16, 126-129
Local Area Networks (LANS), access by disabled, 126, 128, 155

Magnifiers for printed material. *See* CCD's and CCTV's
Morse Code, inputting information, 2, 97-99
  tutorials, 97
Mouse emulation, for input, 84-85
Mouth stick use for data entry, 71-73

National Association for the Visually Handicapped, 8
National Captioning Institute, 113
National Federation for the Blind, 27, 45, 133
National Library service
  braille quality assurance, 40, 43-44, 160-61
  description of services, 8
  statistics, ix, xi, 8, 145
National Technology Center. *See* American Foundation for the Blind

Ohio Library Association, 133
Online catalogs and databases, 115, 126, 155
Optical Character Recognition Systems (OCR),
  basic features, 63
  development of, 63
  requirements for use, 64, 68-69, 163

Packaged adaptive computer systems. *See* Ready-made systems
Paperless braille display, 29-33
Paraplegics and computer access. *See* Interfaces for special entry; Switches; Voice input
Patron training for adaptive technology, 136, 162, 165-66
Personal computers (PCs) and adaptive technology
  need for, ix-x, 1-3, 143
  purchasing equipment, 9-10
Phoenix Public Library Special Needs Center, 115, 118, 127
Physical disabilities. *See also* Keyboard, configurations; Furniture selection for accessibility; Switches; Voice input
  accessing information, 1-2
  adaptions for, 1-3.
  statistics, 6
Pointing systems. *See* Switches, and head control
Public Law 101-43, Television Decoder Circuitry Act of 1990, 112
Public Law 101-336, 42 USC 12101-12212. *See* Americans With Disabilities Act
Puff & Sip entry. *See* Switches, and mouth control
Pushbutton switch entry. *See* Switches, and hand control

Quadraplegics and computer access. *See* Interfaces, for special entry; Switches; Voice input

184 General Index

Ready-made systems, 129-31
Recording for the Blind, ix, 159
Reference materials, special format, ix-x, 154
Ridgewood Public Library, 67, 129
Rocker switches, 1. *See also* Switches, and hand control

SALS (Skokie Accessible Library System Services), 127
Sam S. Miguel Memorial Library, 160
Scanning for computer input, 95-97. *See also* Interfaces, for special entry
Screen magnifiers. *See* Large print, screen displays
Seattle Public Library, 127
Simpson Model 886, sound level monitor, 40, 160-61
Skokie Public Library, 127
Solenoid, 29-30
Staff, sensitivity training, 132-135
 video tapes for, 107, 133
String switch. *See* Switches, and hand control
Switches
 definition of, 88
 need for, 1-3, 88
 and arm control, 92
 and finger control, 92-94
 and hand control, 92-94
 and head control, 94-95
 and mouth control, 89
 and wrist control, 92-94
Synthesizers
 external, 60-62
 internal, 58-61
 requirements, 48-49, 56-57, 62
 software drivers for, 49-56
Synthetic speech
 definition, 48
 features of, 48-49, 62

TTD/TTY
 definition of, 107
 need for, 107,
 language used with, 108
 large print, 110
 models available, 109-110
Touch screen access, 99-101
Trace Research Center, 72, 159

University of Nebraska, 128
University of North Texas, 128
University of Texas, 115

Visual Impairment, 1
 and computers, *see* Large print
 statistics of, 8
Voice input
 need, 101
 use, 101-104
Voice mail for the deaf, 111
Voice recognition, 1, 101-104

Warwick Public Library, 129

Product/Vendor Index

This index is provided to help you quickly research specific products and locate potential vendors of these products.

Accent-PC, 58, 60-61; available from AICOM, 146; L S & S, 150

Accent SA Turbo, 60-61; available from AICOM, 146; L S & S, 150

Access PC Color Systems, 130; available from L S & S, 150

Adaptive Firmware Card, 77, 80-81; available from L S & S, 150; TASH, 152

Aid + Me, 75, 77, 85, 87; available from ComputAbility, 148

Air Cushion Switch, 89; available from ComputAbility, 148; Prentke-Romich, 151; TASH, 152

ALVA, 31-32; available from HumanWare, 149

Apollo, 60-61; available from BIT (Boston Information Technology), 147

Arkenstone, 64-65; available from Arkenstone, 147; Henter-Joyce, 149

Arm Slot, 92; available from DU-IT Control Systems Group, Inc., 149

Arm Slot Control, 92; available from Prentke-Romich, 151

Artic Focus, 16-17; available from Artic Technologies, 147

Artic Visions, 16-17, 50-52; available from Artic Technologies, 147

Audapter, 52, 55, 61; available from L S & S, 150; Personal Data Systems, 150

Big Vue 229-BVC 20, 23-24; available from L S & S, 150

Big Vue 229-BV19SCT-2A, 23; available from L S & S, 150

Big Vue 229-BV13, 23; available from L S & S, 150

Bloorview Minature Keyboard, 79; available from TASH, 152

Braille N' Speak, 32-33, 39; available from E.M. Vitu, 149; L S & S, 150

Braille Home Row Indicators, 28; available from Hoolean, 149; L S & S, 150

Braille KeyTop Kit, 29; available from Data Cal Corp., 148

Breakthru Box, 75, 86-87; available from EKEG, 149

Caption Maker, 113; available from Computer Prompting Corp., 148

CINTEX, 86-87; available from NanoPac, 150

Closed Captioned Decoders, 113; available from American Communications Institute, 147; Potomac Technology, 151; Radio Shack Division of Tandy, 151; Telecommunications for the Deaf, Inc. 152

Product/Vendor Index

COMPU-LENZ, 19-20; available from Ann Morris Enterprises, Incorporated, 147; L S & S, 150

DaDa Entry, 87; available from Designing Aids for Disabled Adults (DADA), 148
Darci Joystick, 83-84; available from WesTest, 152
DecTalk, 58, 66; available from Digital Equipment Corp., 148
Deluxe LP-DOS, 15; available from Celexx Corp, 148; Optelec, 150
Disk Guides, 73-74; available from Prentke-Romich 151; TASH, 152
DragonDictate, 103-04; available from Dragon Systems 148; L S & S, 150
Dual Rocking Switch, 93; available from Prentke-Romich, 151
Duxbury Braille Translator, 37-39; 160 available from Duxbury Systems, 149; L S & S, 150

Easy Action Hand Switch, 94; available from ComputAbility, 148
Easy Listener, 113-14; available from American Communications Institute, 147; Harris Communications, 149; PhoneTTY Inc., 159
Echo PC, 58-59, 61; available from L S & S, 150; Street Electronics, 151; Western Ctr. for Microcomputers Spec., 152
EKEG Expanded Keyboard, 76-77; available from EKEG, 149; Prentke-Romich, 151; TASH, 152

Excellence Reading System, 130; available from L S & S, 150
Expanded Keyboard II, 77, 81; available from ComputAbility, 148
Expanded Membrane Keyboard, 77; Availablle from ComputAbility, 148
Eyegaze, 75, 139; available from LC Technologies, Inc.,150
ezMorse, 98; available from Regenesis Development Corp., 151
ezScan, 96; available from Regenesis Development Corp., 151

4-Pneumatic Switch, 89; available from DU-IT Control Systems Group, Inc., 149; Prentke-Romich, 151; TASH, 152
4-Pushbutton Switch, 92-93; available from TASH, 152; ZYGO, 153
5-Pushbutton Switch, 92-93; available from TASH, 152; ZYGO, 153
5-Thread Switch Slot Control, 92; available from ZYGO, 153
Finger Flex, 94; available from Luminaud, 150
Flex Switch, 94; available from TASH, 152
Flipper, 52-53, 57; available from Omnichron, 150
Footmouse, 85; available from Versatron Corp., 152
Freeboard, 96-97; available from Pointer Systems, 151
FreeWheel, 95; available from Pointer Systems, 151

Gateway, 31; available from TeleSensory Products, Inc., 152

Product/Vendor Index

Gizmo, 17, 162; available from Artic Technologies, 147

HAL, 162-163; available from BIT, 147
HandiCODE, 98; available from Microsystems, 150
HandiKEY, 97; available from Prentke-Romich, 151
Head Switch, 95; available from Luminaud Inc., 150
Headband Switch, 95; available from ComputAbility, 148
HeadMaster, 94-95; available from Prentke-Romich, 151
Headstart III-CD, 130-31; available from Henter-Joyce, 149
Hotdots, 34-36, 125; available from Raised Dots Computing, 151

IBM PC Voice Communication Option, 103; available from IBM Education Systems National Support Center, 149
IBM Phone Communicator, 111; available from IBM Education Systems National Support Center, 149
IBM Screen Reader, 55-57, 59-60; available from IBM Education Systems National Support Center, 149
Index, 40-41; available from Tele-Sensory Products, Inc., 152
InFocus, 14-15; available from A-1 Squared, 146
IntroVoice III, V, VI, 104; available from Voice Connection Products, 152
IRIS, 68; available from VISU-AIDE 2000, Inc., 152

JAWS, 53, 55, 57, 130; available from Henter-Joyce, 149; L S & S, 150

Keyguard, 73; available from ComputAbilitly, 148; COPH-2, 148; Prentke-Romich, 151
Keyport 60, 79-80; available from Polytel Computer Products, 151 Keyport 176, 78; available from Polytel Computer Products, 151 Keyport 300, 77-78; available from Polytel Computer Products, 151
KeyStopers, 73; available from Hoolean Corp, 149; L S & S, 150
KEYUP, 72; available from Ability Systems Corporation, 146
Kurzweil Personal Reader, 66-67; 128-29; available from Xerox-Kurzweil Industries, 153

Left/Right Rocker Switch, 93; available from Don Johnston Developmental Equipment, 148
LIAISON, 99; available from DU-IT Control Systems Group, Inc., 149
LYNX, 21; available from Tele-Sensory Products, Inc., 152

Magnetic FInger Switch, 94; available from Luminaud Inc., 150
MBOSS, 41; available from HumanWare, 149
Memory Printer MP20, MP20D, MP40, 109; available from American Communications Corp., 147; AT & T Special

Needs Center, 147; Harris Communications, 149; Krown Research, 150
Mini-Joystick, 94; available from TASH, Inc., 152
Mini Keyboard, 80; available from ComputAbility, 148
Mini-Rocker Switch, 93; available from Prentke-Romich, 151
MiniCom II, IV, 110; available from UltraTec, 152
Miniprint II, 109; available from American Communications Corp, 109; Harris Communications, 149; Potomac Technology, 151; UltraTec, 152
MorseK, 98; available from Kintetic Designs, 150
Mouse Trak, 85; available from Itac Systems, 150
Multi-Access Package, 96; available from Regenesis Development Corp., 151

Navigator, 31, 124; available from Telesensory Products, Inc., 152
Nomad, 60; available from Syntha-Voice Computers, Inc., 151

1-Key, 71; available from Regenesis Development Corp, 151
Octobraille 84, 31; available from HumanWare, 149
Ohtsuki, 41-43; available from American Thermoform, Inc., 147;
One Finger, 72; available from Trace Center, 152; L S & S, 150
Open and Closed Captioning Software, 113; available from Computer Prompting Corporation, 148
Optelec 20/20, FDR 23, FDR 23C, 22, 24; available from Celexx Corp, 148; Optelec, 150
OsCAR, 68; available from Telesensory Products, Inc., 152

Panorama, 16; available from Syntha-Voice Computers, Inc., 151
PC Braille, 36-37; available from ARTS Computer Products, Inc., 147
PC Drills, 97; available from Personally Developed Software, 151
PC/KPR, 65-66; available from Xerox-Kurzweil Industries, 153
PC Lens, 15; available from ARTS Computer Products, Inc., 147
PC Mini Keyboard, 81; available from TASH, 152
PC Serial AID, 86-87; available from Don Johnston Developmental Equipment, 148; L S & S, 150; TASH, 152
PC-TRAC, 84; available from MicroSpeed, Inc., 150
Penta Switch, 92; available from TASH, 152
Pixelmaster 2, 45-46; available from American Thermaform, Inc., 147, Howtek Incorporated, 149; L S & S, 150
Portaview PV 20+, PV20D, PV20 Jr., 109; available from American Communications Corp., 147; AT & T Special Needs Center, 147; Harris Communications, 149; Krown Research, 150

Product/Vendor Index 189

Powerama, 17; available from Syntha-Voice Computers, Inc., 151
PowerMouse 100, 84; available ProHance Technologies, 151
Prose 4000, 59; available from Centigram Communication Corp., 148
PSS (Personal Speech System), 61-62; available from L S & S, 150; Votrax Inc., 152

Ransley Braille Interface, 39; available from HumanWare, 149; L S & S, 150
Romeo Printer, 44, 161; available from Enabling Technology, 149
Rocker Switch, 93; available from TASH, 152
ScanPac, 96; available from Adaptive Communications Systems, 96
ScanRite, 68-69; available from ATR Computer Tec., 147
ScanWriter, 96; available from ZYGO Industires, 153
SeeBeep, 107, 126; available from Microsystems, 150
SeeTec-STC20, 22-24; available from L S & S Group, 150; Seeing Technologies, 151
Slimware, 59, 163; available from SynthaVoice Computers, Inc., 151
Soft Vista, 15-16; available from TeleSensory Products, Inc., 152 String Switch, 93; available from Ablenet, 146
Superprint 200, 400 TDD, 109-10; available from Krown Research,, 150, L S & S 150, UltraTec, 152

SynPhonix, 59, 61; available from Artic Technologies, 147
Syntha Voice, Model I, 59-61; available from SynthaVoice Computers, 151

Talking Encyclopedia, 131; available from Talking Computer Systems, 152
Thumb Switch, 93; available from ZYGO Industries, 153
Touch System, 100-01; available from Carroll Touch, Inc., 148
TouchWindow, 100; available from Edmark Corporation, 149
Touchware PC Translator, 101; available from Newex, Inc., 151
Turbo Pedal, 50; available from Artic Technologies, 147

Ultimate Reader I, 129; available from L S & S, 150
Ultratec Superprint 100-D-TDD, 110; available from UltraTec, 152
Unicorn Mini Keyboard, 81; available from Prentke-Romich, 151; TASH Inc., 152
Unicorn Expanded Keyboard II, 78-79; available from L S & S, 150; Prentke-Romich, 151; TASH Inc., 152
UNI-PTC, 110; available from American Communications Institute, 147; Integrated Microcomputer Systems, 149; Phone TTY, 151
Unmouse, 101; available from MicroTouch, 150

Vantage CCD, 21, 24; available from TeleSensory Products, Inc., 151
VersaPoint, 40, 43-44, 161; available from Raised Dots Computing, 151; TeleSensory Products, Inc., 151
Voice Master, 104; available from Covox, Inc., 148
Votrax Votalker, 52-53; available from L S & S, 150; Votrax Inc., 152
VoxBox, 55, 61-62; available from Adhoc Reading Systems, 146
Voyager 21, 115, 129; available from TeleSensory Products, Inc., 151

WSKE II, 98-99; available from Adaptive Communications Systems, 146

ZoomText, 13-14, 119-120; available from A-1 Squared, 146

342783

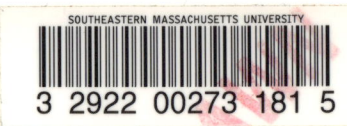